SEX AND SEXUALITY

Dana Lear

SEX AND SEXUALITY

Risk and Relationships in the Age of AIDS

SAGE Publications
International Educational and Professional Publisher
Thousand Oaks   London   New Delhi

For information:

 SAGE Publications, Inc.
2455 Teller Road
Thousand Oaks, California 91320
E-mail: order@sagepub.com

SAGE Publications Ltd.
6 Bonhill Street
London EC2A 4PU
United Kingdom

SAGE Publications India Pvt. Ltd.
M-32 Market
Greater Kailash I
New Delhi 110 048 India

Printed in the United States of America

Library of Congress Cataloging-in-Publication Data

Lear, Dana.
    Sex and sexuality: Risk and relationships in the age of AIDS /
author, Dana Lear.
        p. cm.
    Includes bibliographical references and index.
    ISBN 0-7619-0477-8 (acid-free paper). — ISBN 0-7619-0478-6 (pbk.:
acid-free paper)
        1. College students—California—Sexual behavior. 2. Sex customs
California. 3. AIDS (Disease)—California. I. Title.
HQ27.L43 1997
    306.7—dc21   97-4596
This book is printed on acid-free paper.

97 98 99 00 01 02 03 10 9 8 7 6 5 4 3 2 1

Acquiring Editor:	Peter Labella
Editorial Assistant:	Jessica Crawford
Production Editor:	Sherrise M. Purdum
Production Assistant:	Karen Wiley
Typesetter:	Rebecca Evans
Cover Designer:	Candice Harman

Contents

Preface

This book was originally meant to be about how cultural beliefs influence risk for HIV transmission among Baganda women. I had read everything available in the African press about AIDS. I had spent time in some half dozen countries in West Africa when AIDS was still considered a Western disease, and I wanted to learn about East Africa, where it was already acknowledged as a serious problem. A chance meeting at the International Conference on AIDS in 1989 provided the contact to incorporate "behavioral" research into an established epidemiologic project in Kampala, Uganda. A government invitation was arranged, a Ugandan counterpart identified, all that remained was funding. To my disappointment, funding was not forthcoming; however, the project of which my research was meant to be a part disbanded in what would have been the middle, and so it was fortunate that I had shifted my focus locally. Consequently, this book is about how the cultural beliefs of university students influence their sexuality.

While preparing for the original fieldwork, I had occasion to negotiate the beginning of two sexual relationships. As the mother of a preschooler, doctoral student, community-level worker in women's and sexual health since 1976, I had always been comfortable discussing sexuality. Suddenly, I found it awkward and uncomfortable to be discussing sexual and STD testing histories in terms of my own risk and that of my prospective partners. Steeped in the AIDS public health literature, a member of the San Francisco Women's AIDS Network, I knew it was the "right" thing to do. Sandwiched between the romance of the free love movement of the late 1960s and the power sex and new conservatism of the 1980s, I was a member of the disco generation. We had had several years of sexual liberation and the pill to protect us when I went off to university in the mid-1970s, against the backdrop of my parents' own 1950s consciousness. Yet perhaps because of all this, uncomfortable though it was, discussing one's sexual history was nonetheless possible and even expected among adults in the Berkeley, California, of the 1990s.

Seeking a replacement topic, I began wondering about how the generation of kids leaving home in the early 1990s were dealing with *their* sexual relationships. They were born as I was awakening sexually. Surely, as a product of parents of the 1960s and 1970s, it would be different for them? They would have parents who were open about sex, a wave of feminism that had existed all their lives, HIV and school sex education a fact of their adolescence. The basic questions really didn't seem all that different from the effect of cultural beliefs on sexual mores among the Baganda.

I thought, or perhaps hoped, that sexual desire for them would have been freed from guilt, that some sort of gender equality would have been attained, that homophobia among university students would be nonexistent, that the pressure of HIV might have made open communication and nonlinear sexual goals a normal part of adolescent sexuality.

To my surprise, I was quite wrong. Things have changed, of course, but not nearly as much progress had been made as I had hoped. True, homophobia on the Berkeley campus was slight, but young people still worry about coming out, especially to their families. Condoms are accepted but not entirely without resistance. Young women still worry about their reputations and keeping men, and young men—well, what *do* young men worry about? True to stereotype, heterosexual men especially were a little less aware, a little less proactive. They cared about their partners and their friends, sometimes intensely, but were less interested in process. Feelings were sheltered behind jokes, and barriers stood in the way of intimate relationships, both sexual and nonsexual. The surprise was that *plus ça reste la, plus c'est même chose.*

In spite of barriers to communication with each other, both men and women were as open with me as they could be, for which they have my appreciation. Their participation wasn't tied to any course requirement, and they were scarcely interested in the money they received for their time. I hope their voices are heard here without too much interruption from me. I would also like to thank Bernard

Griego, Cathy Kodama, and Josh Gamson for access to their classes; Carol D'Onofrio, Art Reingold, Judith Warren Little, David Eaton, and Gerard Sullivan for their critical support; my colleagues at the University of Sydney, who gave me the time to finish the book, especially Freidoon Khavarpour and Cherry Russell, and Tim Wong who made good comments and endless trips to the library for me; and Heather and Charlie Yeatman and Toni Schofield for their friendship at the end. The research was partially supported by the University of California, Berkeley's School of Public Health Grossman Fund and University of California, San Francisco's AIDS Clinical Research Center; the final writing was supported in part by a Sydney University School of Community Health research grant.

Finally, I thank Max, born with this project and now 8 years old, who has so often sacrificed time together with equanimity. This work has always been for him.

1

Sexual Negotiation in the Age of AIDS

The advent of AIDS has demanded consideration of the social constructions of risk and trust with respect to sexual negotiation
that has gone beyond fear of HIV itself. Along with HIV, the estab-
lishment of relationships, STD protection, and sexual coercion are
major themes around which sexual negotiation among young adults
occurs. As a public health issue, HIV has become increasingly preva-
lent among youth (Gold, Li, & Kaldor, 1994; Morton, Nelson, Walsh,
Zimmerman, & Coe, 1996), STD rates remain high (Division of STD
Prevention, 1995), and issues of sexual consent and coercion have
been debated vociferously over the past decade. However, it is only
by understanding the processes and contexts involved in negotiating
sexual relationships from the perspective of young people that effective prevention and intervention programs can be designed. To do that,
we must understand the connections among sexuality, gender, relationships, consent, and the perception of risk. This study explores
how sexual communication does and does not occur among young
adults, how gender and sexual orientation influence the ability to
negotiate for safer sex, what strategies are employed for risk reduction, and what barriers to open communication exist. It assumes sexual behavior as a communicative form, both reflective and reflexive,
subject to interpretation that varies according to the participant and
created interactively within and between sexual partners and among

their friends. It further assumes sexuality as a social construction, subject to variance across culture and time (Kitzinger, 1987; Plummer, 1975; Vance, 1984, p. 8).

After briefly discussing the study of sexuality, which follows, Chapter 2 begins by discussing the application of a critical inter-actionist perspective to the study of sexuality. Chapters 3 through 6 continue with the interview results, the methodological focus of this research. Finally, Chapter 7 discusses the findings and their implications for health education research and practice.

Sexual Culture and the Study of Sexuality

Like previous epidemics, HIV is historically situated, confronting global social and cultural systems and posing problems that must be integrated with extant notions of health and sexuality. Like other epidemics, AIDS is more than a medical phenomenon.[1] Although its general prevalence among youth in industrialized countries, such as the United States, Canada, the United Kingdom, and Australia, remains relatively low, its symbolic significance is high. Changing risky behavior because of fear or threat of HIV reduces risk of more common sexually and intravenously transmitted diseases, such as chlamydia, syphilis, and hepatitis. Initiating dialogue among young people about acknowledging desire, the right to request or refuse sex, and negotiating sex can be a positive social effect of HIV prevention programs or conversely, as Frankenberg (1992) points out, can be used to further control and restrict their sexuality. To design effective intervention programs, however, preventive research must explore the construction of HIV within existing explanatory systems, particularly in terms of the symbols, images, and representations that are associated with them (Parker & Carballo, 1990). Meaning and thus social reality are socially negotiated and symbolic because they are mediated through language, symbols, and interaction. Communication is the medium for exploring the complicated relations between behavior and culture, in this case, sexual culture.

Sexual culture consists of the systems of meaning, knowledge, beliefs, and practices that structure sexuality in different social contexts (Parker & Carballo, 1990) and is constructed interactively and collectively. Within the context of sexual culture, notions of risk perception and gendered power relations must be examined, for example, to assess the meaning of condoms in different settings, because social norms may dictate when and with whom contraceptives are used for disease prevention. To understand the meaning of HIV for a particular group, we must understand the construction of sexual identity and sexual behavior, risk and relationships. Similarly, to understand coercion in sexual relationships, we must understand the meaning of consent and resistance. First, let us examine the case of HIV.

THE SOCIAL CONSTRUCTION OF AIDS

The presentation of AIDS as a disease of high risk groups is now well understood as a result of a social process defined by empirical reality that was shaped by ideologies of health and sexuality (Frankenberg, 1994). Like the bubonic plague and syphilis, AIDS has been the site of struggle over not only the disease itself but of what can go wrong in societies in which such epidemics occur (Holland, Ramazanoglu, & Scott, 1990). Public reaction toward AIDS has moved universally in societies through stages of denial, scapegoating, and blame before any constructive response to the epidemic occurs (Lear, 1990). By distancing themselves from identified high risk groups, average people leave their own behavior and notions of risk unchallenged. This distancing from risk leaves populations unprepared to cope with the spread of the epidemic on either personal or national levels. It has also impeded analysis of secular definitions of culture and power with respect to gender and sexuality and given nonsecular interests a platform from which to promote their "family values" agendas.

To offset this politically conservative threat, AIDS activists have worked very hard in the first decade of the epidemic—and were successful to some degree—to emphasize that it is behavior and not individuals that must be avoided. However, neither the activist nor the conservative approaches of the late 1980s and early 1990s left much room for discourse about the nature of trust and risk within intimate relationships or even the distinctions between sexual behavior, sexual identity, and sexual orientation. The epidemic has taught us that people don't necessarily perceive their own behavior as risky nor do they necessarily equate their sexual behavior with their sexual identity. Lever, Kanouse, Rogers, and Hertz (1992) cautioned against using sexual identity rather than sexual behavior as a criterion for risk: in their study of bisexuality, they found that nearly two thirds of the men in their sample who engaged in bisexual behavior as adults identified themselves as heterosexual, implying difficulty for prevention efforts that challenge impression management. It has become a truism that many Latin men in active homosexual roles can still consider themselves heterosexual (Carrier, 1985); conversely, many women engaged in bisexual behavior identify themselves as lesbian (Barkan et al., 1996; Kemp et al., 1993). Both phenomena are constructed within a culture or subculture and carry with them political and social meanings, wherein bisexuals are given lower status than heterosexuals and lesbians, respectively. They may further carry personal meaning where sexual behavior happens to be incongruent with sexual identity, though the latter condition may be a result of the former; that is, if bisexuality were more acceptable socially, perhaps more people would identify with it.

Redefining identity, orientation, behavior, and gender challenges the rigid oppositional thinking embedded in Western thought. Examining sexual practice threatens personal and socially defined categories of acceptable sexual behavior, raises questions about sexual dominance, and challenges predominant ideas about sexual morality (Holland, Ramazanoglu, & Scott, 1990), but it is only by exploring the dialectic of sexual identity and practice that progress can be made in AIDS prevention. We have proceeded with assumptions about the way people behave and with whom they identify that have too often proved incorrect. We don't really know very much, for example, about the impact of feminist praxis on women's personal ability to negotiate sexually or the effect of the AIDS epidemic on young people's personal perceptions of risk or willingness to incorporate condoms, spermicides, or alternate forms of sexual expression into their repertoires.

Social research on AIDS has often been based on epidemiological surveys—usually knowledge, attitude, and practice surveys, although there has been some movement toward using qualitative studies as a prelude to the quantitative. Both approaches to research imply how best to obtain reliable and valid knowledge. At the same time, understanding of the process of negotiation of sexual behavior requires levels of trust and language for which public health has few concepts, making the necessary examination and analysis difficult. There has been political pressure on public health to keep the language of sexuality vague, particularly in the United States, so that there is little information about what behaviors are truly within the realm of normal practice or what shared meanings do exist. Public health has thus far borrowed little from sociological understandings of sexualities, from feminism, critical theory, postmodernism, or queer theory, allowing little benefit from the work in these areas.

SEXUALITY AND ADOLESCENTS: WHY STUDY COLLEGE STUDENTS?

As many researchers have noted, adolescents, and college students in particular, are likely to experiment sexually, often with multiple partners and without using condoms on a regular basis (e.g., Dunne et al., 1994; Hein, 1988; Lucke, 1994; Lucke, Dunne, Donald, & Raphael, 1993; Middleton, Harris, & Hollely, 1994; Moore & Rosenthal, 1993; Office of National AIDS Policy, 1996; White & De-Blassie, 1992). College students are worthy of study in their own right because of their high rates of sexually transmitted disease (Ashcroft, Schlueter, & Thorton, 1991), because problems of date rape on university campuses have been highly publicized, because behavior change tends to diffuse from them to other youth (Yankelovich, 1974), and because they may provide insight that will inform study among less accessible populations. If we agree to look at risk behavior rather than risk groups, college students do indeed warrant attention where they are involved with multiple partners, particularly without knowing each other's serostatus, and where their behavior puts them at risk for coercive sexual encounters (Sanday, 1990). In 1992, the year in which this study began, gonorrhea rates, for example, were 1031.4 per hundred thousand for 15 to 19 year olds and 996.2 for 20 to 24 year olds (Division of STD Prevention, 1995). These rates have since dropped markedly among White youth, perhaps as a result of behavior change due to fear of HIV. Measures that effect change in HIV-related behavior will also affect high rates of other STDs among youth; because of its salience, HIV awareness and behavior change are used as a social indicator for this study. Though the generalized HIV epidemic among young people that was anticipated has not transpired, it was feared and expected in 1992 to 1993 when these interviews took place, an example of the social construction of the epidemic at that moment in time. Lastly, though college students are by no means an oppressed group, they struggle to make sense of issues of gender, identity, sexuality, and their place in the world as other youth do.

ADOLESCENCE TO ADULTHOOD

The college years may be viewed as an extension of adolescence or as a stage in its own right, marked by sexual experimentation and substance use.[2] College students may not have moved far enough beyond adolescence to have abstract future risks override peer pressure and desire for social acceptance in sexual decision making. They straddle a developmental stage between adolescence and adulthood, functioning at once as members of both groups and neither (Roscoe & Peterson, 1984). In their Eriksonian developmental approach to sexual intimacy among men and women in transition between late adolescence and young adulthood, Paul and White (1990) considered most college students still rather egocentric and concerned primarily with social acceptability (p. 378). Communication for them is expressed in general terms, without real understanding or ability to articulate commitment. According to their model, it is only later that sexual partners become capable of empathy, commitment, and communication.

Studies among youth have found that men and women with multiple partners are influenced by their antiprecautionary attitudes in different ways. Interventions must take account of the underlying dynamics according to the type of relationship and behavior that is being addressed. At a time when various media were advising every sex act be protected, Moore and Rosenthal (1991) cautioned that education programs and interventions that underestimated adolescents' abilities to make realistic judgments about risk would be ignored. The moral panic associated with epidemics thus led to overgeneralization based on fear. For example, neither vaginal or anal intercourse nor drug injection objectively posed risk for HIV if both partners were virgins or monogamous and had reliably tested negative or if sterile needles were used and never shared, yet these behaviors were presented as entirely prohibited.

Sexual behaviors that put them at risk for HIV infection are common among adolescents. By the time they are 17 years old, approximately 60% of youth in Canada, the United States, and Australia have had sexual intercourse, usually without condoms or knowledge of each other's HIV serostatus. Only one third of sexually active teenagers uses contraception consistently. Trocki (1992) reported on sexual census data for Northern California's Contra Costa County. In her random sample of 1000 adults, she found the age of sexual debut for those aged 18 to 24 years was slightly past 15 years.

It is a truism that teenagers tend to feel invulnerable, making a future risk of AIDS appear remote. Decisions are thus based on very tangible factors rather than on long-term probabilities (Hein, 1988). One of the milestones that characterizes adolescent psychological development is the ability to incorporate future consequences into current behavior. Peer pressure is an immediate and important factor that can override abstract and distant risks. Thus, friends were expected be a reasonably strong normative influence in this study, and much of the interviews focused on relationships with friends and their opinions and practices.

SEX, GENDER, AND SEXUALITY

Sex here will refer to the biological state of being male or female or to sexual acts, *gender* as applying to socially constructed masculine or feminine role behavior. I am aware that these definitions are currently contested by transgender communities and queer theorists on the basis of a false dichotomy, but I use them here provisionally because they were used thus by study participants. An aim of this study involved defining gender roles with respect to sexual negotiation. Male sexuality is often assumed to be spontaneous and inexorably driven by biological urges, but there has been little qualitative research on how men perceive either their own or women's sexuality nor discussion about how men construct their sexuality in public versus in private. In mainstream Western culture, men are expected to initiate the first sexual encounter, with women deciding how far things will go and being responsible for contraception or refusal (Holland, Ramazanoglu, Scott, Sharpe, & Thomson, 1991a; Leigh, 1989; Wight, 1992).

Many researchers have found that, true to convention, the majority of men might prefer but do not require emotional involvement to have sex, whereas the majority of women will not have sex without it (e.g., Carroll, Volk, & Hyde, 1985; Earle & Perricone, 1986; Gilligan, 1982; Leigh, 1989). Cobliner (1988) discovered that college students are wary of each other: men are afraid of women's emotional needs and demands for time, whereas women fear abandonment, but both sexes are likely to become sexually involved without emotional commitment. Reasons for engaging in sex differ more by sex than sexual orientation, according to Leigh, who found more similarities between lesbians and heterosexual women, and gay men and heterosexual men, respectively.

There is another possibility for explaining reasons for having sex, beyond stereotypical gender role behavior: The conception of the relationship between emotions and sexual desire may be articulated differently by sex. Emotions may be an antecedent, component, or consequence of sexual behavior or some combination of the three. Keller, Elliot, and Gunberg (1982) noted that

> *when normative changes occur in the area of premarital sex, sexual behaviors are likely to change first, followed by changes in sexual attitudes, and finally leading to changes in interpersonal, psychological variables.* If so, we now appear to be between the second and third stage of this "sexual revolution." During the next phase of "consolidation" we can expect to see movement toward uniformity of the sexes on various interpersonal

(power and affiliation) psychological dimensions as they relate to pre-marital sexual relations. (p. 32)

The social reality of AIDS may have an impact on both gender roles and sexuality as little else has by forcing men to be more expressive and women to be more assertive. Before beginning this study, I had expected the university-aged generation following the sexual revolution to have reached the stage of consolidation. It wasn't necessarily so.

Constraints to Communication Among Young People

Adherence to gender roles is only one factor that affects sexual communication. A lack of comprehensive sex education makes communication between partners difficult. The lack of language with which to talk about sexuality, situational factors, and religious background may all influence the ability to negotiate sexually.

EFFECT OF RELIGION ON SEXUALITY

Being raised in a religion is predicted to lead to more conservative sexual behavior and less cautious contraceptive and STD-related behavior because of the inability of a religious adolescent to acknowledge sexual activity (Baldwin, Whiteley, & Baldwin, 1992; Fine, 1988); however, Baldwin et al. found no effect of religious background on sexual activity. White and DeBlassie (1992) noted a substantial inverse correlation between adolescent sexual behavior and religious participation. According to their study, those with an allegiance to the church are more likely to heed its sanctions against sexual activity and to feel more guilt when they don't. Wyatt and Lyons-Rowe (1990, p. 519-522) found that father's educational level, childhood religiousness, and adult religiousness were insignificant with respect to African American women's sexual satisfaction, although childhood church attendance was negatively related. Although these studies suggest mixed and sometimes contradictory effects of religion on sexual behavior and sexual satisfaction, the effect of religious upbringing on sexual communication or negotiation remains uninvestigated.

SEX AND ETHNICITY IN RECENT STUDIES OF AMERICAN YOUTH

Baldwin et al. (1992) noted that studies on U.S. college campuses find that socioeconomic and ethnic variables are not important predictors of sexual behavior. They expected age to affect sexual and contraceptive behavior: older students would be more circumspect in their sexual behavior, use more reliable means of contraception, and use contraception more frequently than younger people. Women would be more conservative in their sexual behavior and more careful in their contraceptive practices than men. Being raised mainly by both original parents was predicted to result in increased conservative sexual behavior.

Baldwin et al. (1992) contended that students' reports of sexual behavior in their study were accurate because they replicated earlier studies (pp. 200-201). They found Asians more sexually conservative than other groups, being significantly less likely than Blacks or Whites to have ever engaged in vaginal and oral sexual relations, and they began vaginal sexual relations about a half year later than Whites. Latinos were significantly less likely to have ever engaged in vaginal and oral sexual relations but used condoms a greater percentage of the time for anal sex, effects that again disappeared when (unspecified) background variables were controlled for. Asians used condoms for vaginal intercourse approximately 10% more of the time than Whites, and African Americans used condoms about 15% more. African Americans also used more effective means of birth control. They found that Latinos used contraception 11.5% less often than other ethnic groups, but the effect disappeared when (unspecified) "mediating" variables were controlled for. Although students had used birth control over 80% of the time, their level of usage left ample room for improvement—perhaps most surprising was the low level of use of spermicide and condoms that protect not only from pregnancy but also from STDs. Spermicide was essentially an ignored means of reducing STD transmission; even the CDC (1993) neither encouraged nor discouraged its use at the time of this study because it considered there were insufficient data to recommend it. Condoms were used an average of 31.1% of the time during vaginal intercourse in the prior 3 months of Baldwin et al.'s (1992) study, up from 23% in an earlier study. Women did have fewer partners than men; older students had fewer per year than younger students. Socioeconomic variables showed little effect on sexual behavior, but they were slightly correlated with increased sexual liberalness and decreased sexual caution.

Huang and Uba (1992) studied UC Berkeley students in 1982. Like Baldwin, they excluded data from gay and married students. They found that levels of sexual experience reported by this sample differed greatly from those reported by studies of non-Chinese-

Americans. The number (40%) of Chinese American college students at UC Berkeley who had engaged in premarital intercourse was much lower (73%-83%) than the number of Caucasian students found in the other studies they cited. In addition, Chinese American women and men were older when they first engaged in sexual intercourse, compared to Caucasian and African American college students (but much younger than Chinese in China): The mean age for first experiencing coitus in their sample was 18.45 years and 18.84 years for Chinese women and men, respectively, whereas the mean age has been reported to be 17.69 years and 16.93 years for Caucasian women and men, respectively, and 16.2 years for African American women. Chinese students in their sample heavily weighed the amount of emotional commitment in deciding what degree of sexual activity was permissible, postponing intimacy longer than their Caucasian counterparts. The authors concluded that approximately one third of male and female Chinese students disapproved of casual sex, which they defined as a "no affection" situation, implying something more prosaic than sex with a noncommitted partner.

Padilla and O'Grady (1987, p. 7) found Mexican American University of California students in Southern California significantly more conservative than Anglo students on measures of autoeroticism, heterosexual relations, and abortion. Women were more conservative than men concerning abortion, and both were more likely to endorse sexual myths and have less sexual knowledge. They found Mexican Americans less sexually experienced, more likely to use condoms, and less likely to use oral contraceptives than European Americans. Mexican American men were more sexually experienced than women (in contrast to Chinese American students), including more likely to have engaged in same-sex behavior.

Theory, Method, and the Study of Sexuality

This section will discuss the difficulties inherent in studying sexuality and the merits of a constructivist perspective in public health research. As an example of such an approach, I will review the epistemological and methodological precepts of constructivist approaches to sexuality, especially interactionist perspectives. I will not discuss Kraft-Ebbing, Kinsey, or Masters and Johnson in this chapter; for comprehensive reviews of sex research, readers are referred to Weeks (1985, and in Caplan, 1987) or Parker and Gagnon (1995). This section will focus on research specifically within the context of the HIV epidemic.

Studying Sex

THE POSITIVIST ACCOUNT

Scientific research has not been immune from the political and moral stances of its practitioners, yet AIDS as a disease has engendered a legitimate forum for the discussion of sexuality that was available to psychology in the form of sexology but hitherto largely unexamined in public health. Abramson (1990) was among the first to discuss research on sexuality within the context of the AIDS epidemic, albeit from the firmly positivist psychological perspective congruent with the epidemiological research carried out in its first years. He believed that to be recognized as real science, research in sexuality must strive to develop concepts and theories that use methods consistent with the objectives of so-called basic science. Abramson maintained that data on demography and sexual practices of gay men that would have advanced epidemiological knowledge at the start of the AIDS epidemic did not exist because the study of sexuality had been devalued and hence underfunded since the time of Kinsey, and the view of homosexuality as pathological and its attendant stigma would have reduced the validity of such research as might have been done. Once bodies such as the World Health Organization, the National Statistical Society, and the National Research Council deemed sexuality a worthy area of study, and biomedical journals such as *Science, Nature, Lancet,* and *The New England Journal of Medicine* commonly began to publish articles on intimate and hitherto unexamined topics, a variety of subjects and methods opened for discussion. As sexually related issues have demanded urgent understanding and action, it has become increasingly important to have an established corpus from which to draw that extends beyond traditional public health perspectives.

Qualitative methods have a place in establishing a foundation of knowledge from which other kinds of scientific endeavors may depart. Abramson (1990) finally acknowledges that sexual science must encourage a wide variety of research methods, including narrative and qualitative assessment and theoretical strategies (pp. 161-162), although nonetheless cautioning that sex researchers remember that "science" is defined by its methods. He warns that if sexual science is to be perceived as a legitimate science, it must use methods that are generally deemed scientific. Qualitative methods, Abramson admits, however, are useful in exploring "sexual variables" that are not easily counted or physiologically measured (p. 155). As a psychologist,

Abramson's training has been very much aligned with the positivist model. Social science may learn more if it draws from anthropological and sociological ways of studying and understanding the world.

SEXUALITY AS A RESEARCH PROBLEM

At the same time as Abramson argued for a legitimate sexual science, Parker and Carballo (1990) argued that there was a lack of "established tradition of theory and method for conducting research on human sexuality," which

> has left AIDS researchers with little or no foundation for the assessment of sexual practices relevant to the spread of HIV infection and has limited their ability to contribute significantly to more effective strategies for AIDS prevention. . . . As important as [survey research is] it has become increasingly apparent that most quantitative surveys of sexual behavior have offered only limited insights into the complex range of social and cultural meanings that may be associated with different behaviors—and to the ways in which behavior itself is shaped by such meanings in different social and cultural settings. (p. 78)

Behavioral research is needed to help explore and explain sexual behavior in ways that can influence behavior change and policy (Rowe, 1996). By situating behavioral data within a wider social and cultural context, qualitative research can potentially offer an important framework for the comparative analysis of data on sexual conduct. Whether carried out in conjunction with quantitative survey research or developed as an end in and of itself, a constructivist approach provides a depth of knowledge and understanding that will ultimately be necessary to develop more effective responses to the risks posed by AIDS. Qualitative methods can contribute to the creation of language that articulates what we are trying to assess. Anthropology has long been concerned with the study of identifying valid category terms within a culture, and we can use that knowledge to develop qualitative methods that will work for public health.

Survey data will lack validity if such research does not precede it. Most surveys have taken the form of knowledge, attitude, and practice (KAP) questionnaires, which have methodological problems with assessments of sexual practice and unsafe sex. Researchers who do not take into account respondents' knowledge of their partners' sexual history and HIV antibody status and their meaning for sexual actors may incorrectly categorize all unprotected intercourse as risky behavior, as Gaies, Sacco, and Becker (1991) do. Furthermore, many fixed-choice questionnaires ask questions such as "Have you changed your behavior because of AIDS?" A person who has undergone a behavior change that was not a direct response to HIV (involuntary celibacy, for example) would have to answer in the negative and might be incorrectly scored as at risk and not responding to education efforts, as in Roscoe and Kruger (1990). A questionnaire asking "How often do you use condoms when having sex with someone who is not a regular partner?" as James, Bignell, and Gillies (1991) do, might get a response of "never" from a woman involved in a lesbian relationship, who might then be scored as high risk. A couple that has tested together and believes in each other's monogamy would not consider themselves at risk, and might indeed not be at risk, but would nonetheless similarly be assessed as at risk. In their survey of high school virgins, Schuster, Bell, and Kanouse (1996) warn us of the risk behavior of young people who engage in oral sex without asking whether their partners might also be virgins. Thus, KAP and other fixed-choice surveys are limited in their contribution to understanding how people understand their sexual relationships.

Abramson (1990) noted that, as sexually related issues demanded urgent understanding and action, it became increasingly important to have an established corpus from which to draw. However, the quantitative measurement of sexual behavior he recommended carried the risk of treating aspects of sexuality as a social or medical problem although ignoring the meaning and importance of sexuality in people's lives. He acknowledged, finally, that sexual science must encourage a wide variety of research methods, including narrative and qualitative assessment and theoretical strategies (pp. 161-162), all the while maintaining what Foucault (1980, p. 51) referred to as "the rarefied and neutral viewpoint of a science." The validity of an objective stance in social science research has been argued extensively elsewhere and will not be repeated here, but Abramson's view was useful at the time to bridge the chasm between researchers mapping epidemiological patterns and those more interested in the meanings of the behaviors under investigation.

Contribution of This Study

Prior research had really not examined the construction of HIV within the existing explanatory systems of college students nor addressed how they responded to the presentation of AIDS as a gay disease in light of their own risk behaviors. Furthermore, many are still at risk for date rape, sexually transmitted HIV, and other sexually transmitted diseases because of their sexual behavior. By deconstructing risk and its inverse, trust, we can better understand how to approach prevention with this group.

Little work has been done that examines the sexual categories that are present or absent among young adults or the effects of these categories on precautionary behavior. How does the definition of sex affect risk avoidance, and under what circumstances does it vary? How does the type of relationship affect the precautionary strategies employed? Have the feminist movement or the HIV epidemic had an impact on the construction of sexual identity or on individuals' ability to articulate their desires or negotiate sexually? This study examined how men and women perceive their own and their partners' sexual agency within the contexts of consensual sexual encounters. It also investigated experiences with coercive sex and their impact on risk behavior and the ability to negotiate sexually afterward, another topic about which we have little information. At the time this work was undertaken, only Fine (1988) and the Women Risk and AIDS Project (Holland, Ramazanoglu, Scott, Sharpe, & Thomson, 1990; Holland, Ramazanoglu, Scott, Sharpe, & Thompson, 1991; Holland, Ramazanoglu, Sharpe, & Thomson, 1991) had published research with young people that explored the meaning of sexual negotiation among them.

Separation of research participants by sexual orientation in previous studies has created artificial distinctions that may obscure the effect of gender and moreover, further contribute to the marginalization of lesbian, gay, and bisexual youth. This study explored the effect of gender roles on sexual negotiation, combining individuals with varying sexual orientations to determine whether gender role might have greater impact than sexual orientation on sexual negotiation. Interviews included questions about ethnicity, class background, and religiosity, but these themes did not prove important for most participants, though exceptions are noted. By approaching issues of risk from an interactionist perspective, this study contributes to a greater understanding of sexuality and how issues of sexual negotiation relate to sexual identity and sexual relationships.

Notes

1. See, of course, Camus' *The Plague* for the classic treatment of the social side of epidemics. The ebola fever outbreak in Zaire in the mid-1990s was only the most recent example of the ways in which viruses threaten peoples' notions of safety in ways that do not necessarily correspond to their actual risk.

2. Adolescence is variously defined as the period beginning somewhere between age 11 and 13 years and ending between 17 and 22 years. Gordon (1996) mentions a definition in which adolescence ends when a person is physically mature, socially and economically independent, and capable of "mutuality in relationships" (p. 889). University students particularly push the later boundary of adolescence because of their delayed financial independence. Because the issues presented in the literature have been so similar, for the purposes of this book, it will be assumed that adolescence is similar enough among anglophone Western industrialized countries (i.e., the United States, Canada, the United Kingdom and Australia) to generalize among them. At the time of this writing, I am working on two follow-up studies in Australia to see whether they are indeed equivalent.

2

The Social Construction of Sexuality

Theory and Method in AIDS Prevention

The future of public health education arguably lies in its ability to make itself meaningful to everyone concerned in as culturally appropriate and specific a way as possible. The aim, therefore, may not be generalizability but transferability, for it is my contention that any particular health education endeavor should be at once universal and specific and as such, should reflect the particular and peculiar concerns of those for whom the intervention is intended. Although it is important to educate the population about general health risks, a grand health education is as reductionist as any grand theory and thereby rendered ultimately irrelevant. With this in mind, researchers are applying microsociological and psychological theories to AIDS prevention.

Leviton (1989) divided theories current in health education that may be applied to AIDS prevention into categories addressing cognitive approaches, fear arousal, interpersonal relations, and communication and persuasion. Variants of the Health Belief Model (Rosenstock, 1974) and Prochaska and DiClemente's Stages of Change (e.g., Grimley, Prochaska, Velicer, Blais, & DiClemente, 1994) have become popular in HIV education programs because both address self-efficacy and barriers to change. Symbolic interactionism as a social psychological theory has been employed to explore both health and sexuality (Becker, 1961; Glaser & Strauss, 1971; Goffman, 1961; Plummer, 1975). However, interactionism has not been widely used in health education research, and only Levine (1992), Spigner (1989-1990), and Taylor and Lourea (1992) have used it to understand HIV. Levine recommended it to frame discourse on homosexuality; Spigner has used it to make recommendations for its use in prevention programs among African Americans; Taylor and Lourea used Goffman's dramaturgical analysis to suggest a framework for incorporating safer sex behaviors among gay men; Ulin (1992) has suggested its use in AIDS prevention research in Africa. Though the need was recognized (e.g., Gagnon, 1992), until very recently, little attention was given in mass education efforts to the differences in social worlds of gay men or young African Americans in San Francisco, IV drug injectors in New York, married women in Kigali, and university students in Berkeley, yet each indicates great differences in prevention needs. Sexual behavior, for the purposes of AIDS education, was long regarded as either heterosexual or homosexual, thus ignoring the range of sexualities recognized in Brazil (see Parker, 1992) and the same-sex practices throughout the world that are considered heterosexual. To create AIDS education that works, first we must have an accurate idea not only of a taxonomy of behaviors that pose risk but also how they are regarded in the cultural context to be addressed and what interactional forces shape and sustain them. The methods of choice for investigating such meanings are naturalistic (Denzin, 1971), or qualitative, and will be discussed as they apply to the current study.

Social Constructivist Approaches and the Study of Sexuality

Various tensions continue among approaches to sexual health: between public health and the biological sciences, between epidemiology and health promotion, between research and intervention, between quantitative and qualitative methods. Research on the transmission dynamics of HIV has helped to legitimize the study of sexual behavior and contributed to a dialogue on the nature of good science, the purpose of research in public health, and the appropriate methods for studying sexuality. AIDS was presented and claimed by the biomedical model, and it was this model that has largely defined the discourse of the epidemic (Gagnon, 1992). Though biomedical perspectives on sexuality have been and continue to be contested by postmodernists and constructivists (notably by Foucault, 1980, 1984; Gagnon, 1977; and Gagnon & Simon, 1973), feminists and queer theorists, the very fact that they challenge the hegemonic position denotes their historically less privileged stance in the debate. Within a public health perspective, these challenges offer valuable balance between examining sexual practice and exploring its meaning to sexual partners; hence, this work sits somewhat uneasily between positivist and postmodern perspectives as an interactionist approach framed by a feminist perspective.

Public health was not the only field of study unprepared to deal with HIV. Even anthropology, with its claim to categorizing sexual customs and mores, was reluctant to regard sexuality as a legitimate subject of study (Vance, 1991) until the early 1990s. By 1991, Parker, Herdt, and Carballo (1991) stressed the importance of an understanding of the meaningful context in which sexual behavior takes place and the subjective meaning that this interaction invests in such behavior for individuals. By focusing on meaning, it is possible to address a range of issues related to the significance of sexual behavior: its erotic and social values, what makes a particular sex act or partnership satisfying, its psychological impact, and so on. Nuanced understandings of the meanings associated with sexual behavior, with criteria for partner selection and notions of desire and pleasure, have only recently become a focus of research in relation to HIV and should also be applied to other situations of sexual risk, such as sexually transmitted diseases and coercive sexual encounters (Parker & Gagnon, 1995, p. 15). This understanding is critical to translate social and behavioral research findings into more effective prevention strategies. Interpretive interactionism, based on symbolic interactionism, offers a useful theoretical framework with which to explore sexual issues.

Symbolic Interactionism and the Study of Sexuality

Because sexual relationships, like language, are invested with a great deal of symbolic meaning, symbolic interaction can offer a useful framework for the interpretation and understanding of sexuality. Language becomes the medium of study because direct observation is impracticable. Individual lines of action are worked out among persons when they communicate their desires and intentions among themselves. People act on the bases of these communicated meanings—they conduct themselves partly by communicating their own intentions to themselves and partly by observing the adjustments made by others to the intentions they have communicated (Skidmore, 1979). Spoken language has been the form most often analyzed, but because sex is a form of communication in a similar sense, its meaning can be studied in reported form. Sexual storytelling, according to Plummer (1995), who also situates his work within an interactionist framework, recounts "the narratives of intimate life, focused especially around the erotic, the gendered and the relational," and has a history dating back at least to Rousseau (pp. 5-6). Symbolic interaction and its descendants, to which I will here collectively refer as *interactionism*, are useful as a theoretical framework to address the intersection of communication, sexual behavior, culture, and the negotiation among them. Sex is a physical act with symbolic meaning that occurs through verbal and nonverbal communication; symbolic interactionism has frequently addressed language and communication and thus may be useful in studying the language of sexuality and its negotiation. Surprisingly few studies have suggested its use to analyze sex (e.g., Ulin, 1992), perhaps because of the difficulty involved in using self report. It therefore has the potential to contribute to an understanding of HIV/AIDS, date rape, and reproductive health issues by leading us to understand the meaning of sexuality within its social context in order to approach prevention.

PHILOSOPHICAL BACKGROUND

Interactionism strives to understand human events as the participants would. Although an observer might use different language to describe behavior and feelings, the general intent is to discover the individual's predicament and situation as he or she sees it. The researcher in this approach lends an additional overview of the situation, knowledge of structural forces or constraints, and a broader vision with which to make comparisons. This knowledge can be combined to describe the social world of a person as a developing process influenced by individuality and institutions, morality and mores (Skidmore, 1979).

Symbolic interaction as described by George Herbert Mead (1934) and articulated by Herbert Blumer (1969) presupposes an interpretive paradigm, wherein research and theory are inextricably linked; its strength "derives in large part from the enormous body of research that embodies and gives meaning to its abstract propositions" (McCall & Wittner, 1990, p. 4). The influences of the Pragmatists led to the interactionist view of society as the continually created product and process of social interaction assuming multiple realities, a subjective epistemology, and naturalistic methodologies. Like Paul Abramson, Mead advocated the use of scientific method as a means of achieving empirical understanding; for him, constructivism was a scientific way of learning about the world. The reader is referred to Denzin (1992) for a thorough review of symbolic interactionism's historical roots.

The language of the theater has been borrowed by interactionists, notably Erving Goffman (1961), with its stage-front and backstage action, roles enacted by significant players, and scenes and presentation to be interpreted and managed. Empirical work is often concerned with the meaning of meaning, which is constructed in the process of interaction. Much of the original interactionist work took place in the early years of the departments of philosophy and sociology at the University of Chicago, where it was recognized that social theory must be based on communication theory. Language is viewed as the instrument of social cooperation and mutual participation, and meaning is achieved through communication. The data of communication are the expressive forms used in social relations; methods help to analyze the forms in which communication occurred. Social behavior is characterized by attempts at impression management in various contexts. Incorporating cultural theory by viewing social practices, relations, and representations as communication and analyzing their construction and reproduction, interactionism maintains a critical stance (Denzin, 1992).

INTERACTIONIST UNDERSTANDING

Interactionist understanding separates the perception of the individual from the social context. Reality is understood through social interaction. Meaning is socially negotiated and symbolic because it is mediated through language, symbols, and interaction. People acquire their self-concepts and learn to attach meaning to their actions through interaction with others. Symbolic interactionism emphasizes the process through which people mutually emit and interpret each other's verbal and physical gestures. From the information gained through this interpretation of gesture, they are able to act and react in the world (Blumer, 1969).

Interactionism involves certain specific processes, the most important of which is that people can objectify themselves and others. The self is viewed as both one's essential being and simultaneously, that which reacts to the gestures of others, the *I* and *me* according to Mead (1982). Norms and values are also objects that guide interaction, existing as referents, which in interactionist terms are the internalized expectations resulting from experience in interaction. Because people act toward objects, it is necessary to understand the world of objects they have symbolically designated. Theoretical understanding thus emerges *from* the data; it does not serve as a framework through which data are collected. I propose that it is a lack of understanding and consensus about the world of objects among individuals and groups that has caused much of health education generally, and AIDS education particularly, to fail.

INDIVIDUAL, COMMUNITY, AND SOCIAL RELATIONS

Microsociological approaches, such as interactionism, are concerned with two principle considerations. The first is what is meant by everyday life; the second is how one goes about studying it, the language one uses to describe it, and the conceptual and methodological focus (Schwartz & Jacobs, 1979). By *everyday life*, symbolic interactionists mean a collection of *places* located in social time and space. That is, they study collections of people in conjunction with settings, activities, and problems that they all face and that make them a group—in this case, young adults. We would ask what the world looks like to university students and use this information to explain their actions and interactions. Symbolic interactionism tries to identify emotions, purposes, and motives that people really have and that determine what they really do and how they do it (Schwartz & Jacobs, 1979), so interpersonal interaction is regarded as the locus of interest.

A fundamental theoretical concern is the attempt to understand how one is able to take the perspective of another in interaction. For example, in symbolic interaction, gendered behaviors are socially prescribed acts acquired—and required—as children become integrated as members of society (Deegan & Hill, 1987). Women and men are viewed as social products who emerge from a process of human interaction based on material and symbolic language and behavior and the human capacity to understand them. Definitions of sexuality and gendered behavior are codified through the actions and shared meanings of large groups of people. An interactionist approach to sexual behavior would thus look at the ordinary human relationships involved in its negotiation and consider the forces that shape and sustain it, thus offering a potential framework for informed intervention at the level at which the behavior occurs. Thus interactionism takes account of larger structures and ideologies in personal relationships.

Symbolic interaction, with its assumption of human flexibility and creativity, points to ways in which individuals can change the group and the community, all levels that must be addressed simultaneously in AIDS prevention, because women, particularly, do not have all the freedom they need to negotiate change in sexual or gender relations. For although symbolic interactionists believe that people create their own lives, this does not mean that change occurs without resistance, trial and error, or ambiguity. Changing the inequality that permeates society requires that those without power gain more power, legitimacy, and control. A large enough number must want change, agree on definitions of what is desirable, and have access to the means to attain these goals (Deegan & Hill, 1987). This is not an easy prospect in response to potential HIV infection among university students who do not perceive themselves at risk or women who must contest the power structure in relationships to demand safety.

The researcher in all this is in a place within the system analogous to that of the participants. To understand the action, the researcher must gain from it the meanings being communicated among the participants. Method, then, becomes "the means of acting on the symbolic environment and making those actions consensual in the broader community of researchers" (Denzin, 1989, p. 14). Denzin extended an approach to interactionism in a way that not only provides understanding but is intended to be applied to social problems.

INTERPRETIVE INTERACTIONISM

Norman Denzin (1978, 1989; Denzin & Lincoln, 1994), currently the primary bearer of the interactionist flame, outlines methodological principles for research. The first is that symbols and interaction must be brought together to make explicit the connection between attitudes and behavior as well as situating them within the social context (Denzin, 1992). The second is that because symbols contribute to attitudes, the reflective nature of the self must be considered. The researcher must take the role of the actor by learning the language and the culture but be able to situate the actor's perspective within the analytical framework of the researcher. Comparability is achieved by revealing as much as possible of the methods used for investigation as well as providing detailed description of individuals as they account for themselves and their interaction. By situating the interaction, even simply by asking in what circumstances a behavior occurs, replication is allowed. Third, and probably most important to Denzin, contemporary interactionist research must include a political critique of the social, gender, racial, and economic forces that shape actors' situations (Denzin, 1992).

Naturalistic methods (i.e., those located in the natural worlds of everyday social interaction) are usually favored over experiments or surveys as a means to interpretive research (Denzin, 1989). Though fieldwork over extended periods serves to minimize the observer effect and is therefore preferred, it may not always be practical in public health research. In interactionist terms, the research itself is seen as an interactive process, wherein the researcher mediates between those being investigated and the research community.

Interactionist interpretation relies on analytic induction, a strategy of analysis that is meant to generate universal propositions through an exhaustive examination of cases in an attempt at theoretical generalization. It involves starting with a theory about some phenomenon, formulating hypotheses as data are collected and simultaneously analyzed, determining whether a case fits the hypothesis, and reformulating the hypothesis as needed until explanation is complete. The latter process, particularly, is not acceptable in the scientific method, where hypotheses are normally accepted or rejected once tested. Those who practice research from an interactionist perspective maintain that triangulation and analytic induction solve most problems of rigor (Vidich & Lyman, 1994). Denzin (1989) has now updated this methodological stance through the development of "interpretive interactionism," which relies on a mutual deconstruction and reframing of the issues between researcher and researched, within a framework of critical understanding of their essential elements within their social and historical contexts.

In *Symbolic Interactionism and Cultural Studies* (1992) and the research annual *Studies in Symbolic Interactionism*, of which he is the editor, Denzin incorporates feminist theory, cultural studies, and communications theory to address some of the historical weaknesses of symbolic interaction. In this way, interactionism offers promise for health education as it becomes more applied and action oriented. Cultural studies contribute by offering a critical appraisal of how "interacting individuals connect their lived experience with the cultural representation of those experiences" (Schwant, 1994, p. 125), whereas feminism provides a perspective for analyzing the social construction of gender and the relationship between researcher and researched (Denzin & Lincoln, 1994).

Feminist theory, like interactionism, recognizes the participatory role of the researcher, where the researcher may disclose details of his or her own life in a conversation that serves to balance the power relation of the research situation (Oakley, 1981). By situating the construction of meaning within the communication process and the larger culture as represented by mass media, one may more easily understand the process whereby AIDS became so firmly established as a disease of the Other. Interpretive interactionism assumes that the perspectives and experiences of those served by the interventions must be grasped, interpreted, and understood if solid, effective programs are to be created. By carefully revealing the researcher's stance as well as critically presenting the lives of the researched (Fine, 1994), interaction and feminism engage in an activist and ethical stance.

BEYOND KNOWLEDGE, ATTITUDE, AND PRACTICE (KAP) STUDIES:
THE NEED FOR QUALITATIVE RESEARCH ON SEXUALITY

Many authors have now commented on the limitations of KAP studies for understanding the meaning of sexual behavior. On reading journal articles based on knowledge, attitude, and practice research, many questions remained for me. For example, in their article concerning contraception and STD prevention among college students, Grimley, Riley, Bellis, and Prochaska (1993) had students respond to a Likert-type statement regarding their contraceptive and condom use. Heterosexually active respondents were asked to indicate whether they had used or intended to use condoms/contraceptives with every sexual encounter. The authors indicated that one student replied that she did not use condoms with her partner because each was the other's first and only partner. Apart from that one explanatory instance, I was left wondering about the "noncompliers," those whom the authors identified as at greater risk for unintended pregnancy: For those who did not use contraception with every act of vaginal intercourse, were they using natural family planning or some other method of indicating nonfertility? What were students' explanations for the perceived or real need to use condoms or not; for example, by what methods was risk established or trust constructed? Such data are best obtained by use of qualitative methods to achieve the theoretical goal of the research, that is, intervention aimed at the appropriate target population and stage of change. This study attempts to address the gap left by survey research.

The dearth of existing research on sexuality warrants qualitative approaches to establish a foundation for evaluating sexual practices by situating them within their social and cultural contexts (Abramson & Herdt, 1990; Herdt & Lindenbaum, 1992; Parker & Carballo, 1990).

Qualitative approaches to the study of HIV have been concerned with discovery of culturally sensitive categories of HIV knowledge, attitudes, and practices in prevention efforts (Herdt & Boxer, 1991). The aim of such approaches is to elicit and study culturally and linguistically sensitive taxonomies of sexuality.[1] Cross-cultural research suggests a wide range of definitions of "sex"; among participants in this study, "sex" usually meant vaginal intercourse between heterosexual partners, oral or anal intercourse between gay men, and orgasm-intended activity between women. Herdt and Boxer note that the variations emphasize the necessity of understanding cultural category distinctions in assessing HIV sexual risk (p. 172).

Qualitative methods may provide sensitive information that cannot be uncovered in surveys or structured interviews and may be used as an end to themselves or to further inform these other methods—for example, where behavior might escape a survey instrument. The rapport possible in a qualitative interview is conducive to more accurate reporting of intimate experience, providing data not available in any other way, and offering validity checks on the interpretation of quantitative data. Qualitative methods can be used to understand the implicit meanings that are often embedded in behavioral patterns—and that may prove crucial to behavioral change (Parker & Carballo, 1990). Though Bolton (1992) argues for the relevance and necessity of participant observation in a radical and disputably courageous way, he also acknowledges its limitations and the difficulty of funding it. Qualitative methods in understanding meaning and behavior related to HIV will normally include in-depth interviews, nonparticipant observation, or both.

Qualitative approaches are meant to complement rather than supplant epidemiological approaches. Where epidemiological methods may provide breadth, qualitative methods offer depth. The notable weakness of qualitative methods may be that the findings of any single study are insufficient to generalize on certain topics. Data might be more easily interpreted among studies if they address three major areas, according to Parker & Carballo (1990): (a) the social context of sexual conduct, (b) the documentation of sexual practice, and (c) the interpretation of behavioral change. Comparability is further enhanced when a qualitative study uses a similar group of participants as existing surveys. In this case, participants in this study are similar to those of Baldwin et al. (1992) whose sample comprised University of California (UC), Santa Barbara students, and to those of Huang and Uba (1992), with UC Berkeley students.

Design of This Study

This study sought to explore how late adolescents-young adults negotiate sexual relationships, how they construct risk, and whether specific demographic variables and life experiences might contribute to risk for HIV or date rape. The primary method employed was in-depth interviews, which were supplemented with questionnaires, analysis of secondary sources, and informal interviews with various university officials. The Appendix describes my position and the methods used in detail.

As an adjunct to the interviews, I administered a questionnaire. The Risk Assessment Questionnaire (RAQ) (Lear, 1994), is a three-page questionnaire designed to explore whether characteristics such as ethnicity, religiosity, and age of parents might be related to sexual history and whether factors such as history of sexual abuse or intra-relationship violence might have a relationship with unsafe sexual practice. It also asked about current and past relationships, recreational drug and alcohol use, and experience with pregnancy and STDs. It was distributed to two health education classes, a sociology of sexuality class, and to interview participants. The RAQ was intended primarily to inform the interviews and is discussed in more detail in the Appendix; results from interviews will be presented in the next chapters.

SAMPLING CONSIDERATIONS

Most studies differentiate between married and unmarried individuals and among heterosexuals, bisexuals, and homosexuals. For example, Moore and Rosenthal (1991) chose to study only heterosexuals among the college students they selected

> because this is the majority group, and the dynamics of AIDS precautionary behavior within this group are largely unknown. These dynamics are likely to be different from those of the more widely studied gay population, for whom there has been a greater apparent acceptance of risk and consequent behavior change. (p. 213)

Moore and Rosenthal (1991) seemed to assume that gay youth have more in common with middle-aged gay men than with other youth; lesbians were not even worthy of note. Much research with gay youth has focused on runaways and other troubled youth (e.g., Pennbridge, Freese, & MacKenzie, 1992; Rotheram-Borus, Meyer-Bahlbur, Rosario, & Koopman, 1992), but little research has been conducted with young gay people without such complicated problems. I disagree with Moore and Rosenthal: little is known about average gay youth and less still about lesbians and lesbian youth. I contend that we should not assume that young gay men have absorbed information about AIDS and behavior change in the same way as middle-aged gay men have done; rather, there has been evidence to the contrary (e.g., Gold & Skinner, 1992). It is important to find out about various sexualities within a similar context, because young gay men, lesbians, and bisexuals may have more in common with heterosexuals of their age and gender than with their older counterparts. Information about bisexuals is especially unknown and problematic because of the secrecy involved and the risk that clandestine behavior poses to uninformed partners. Straight women and lesbians might be expected to be less likely to want to have sex with bisexual men and women, respectively, because of the risk of infection from men, contradicting a common representation of women as reservoir. This study explored the notion that men and women have more in common by sex than by sexual orientation, that gender has a stronger influence on sexual behavior and ability to negotiate sexually than sexual orientation.

UC Berkeley students are the most ethnically diverse university students in the United States. In this study, I attempted to interview students of a range of ethnic backgrounds; participants largely matched those of letters and science undergraduates as a whole. In addition to diversity of gender, sexual orientation, and ethnicity, I looked for a range across the undergraduate years. A tabular description of participants can be found in the appendix on pages 172-173.[2]

Study participants and questionnaire respondents were recruited from undergraduate classes in health and sexuality. Those who participated in interviews were somewhat more experienced sexually, less often heterosexual, and less likely to be virgins than respondents. Survey respondents had a wider range of number of drinks per week than participants and experimented more with recreational drugs. On other measures, such as ethnic background, parents' age, experience of relationship violence, history of sexually transmitted disease, and acquaintance with an HIV+ person, groups were comparable.

The next chapters review the themes that emerged from the in-depth interviews in three parts. First was the normative influences of family, school, and friends regarding sexuality. Second, understanding how romantic relationships were negotiated among these students provides a context for understanding how trust and risk are constructed. It explores how strategies for risk reduction, attitudes

3

Family and Friends

$\mathbf{P}$articipants in this study were children of the 1970s, a time of feminist resurgence and new openness about sexuality. I thought parents might have been easier and more positive about teenage sexuality than previous generations. I thought family and school would be important influences on sexual attitudes and behavior, and possibly on the ability to negotiate sexually, because they are the accepted settings for learning about sex. I was wrong. Most parents weren't particularly more progressive than those of previous generations, and they didn't have more explicit or frank discussions with their children. For study participants, friends were a far greater influence on sexual matters, beginning in the high school years. This chapter reviews sex education in the home and at school, how sex is dealt with among friends, and the impact of university life and drinking on sexual negotiation and behavior.

Sex Education

FAMILY ATTITUDES TOWARD SEX

Interviews explored the experience of family-based and school-based sex education among participants and how they perceived its effectiveness. It happened that students' family background and education had little impact on their sexual behavior. In virtually all cases, parents had not established a pattern of open communication about sexuality; advice about sex was usually limited to a vague warning to be careful. Given the lack of foundation for discussion about sex, by the time parents became willing and attempted to discuss the issue, young people themselves were often reticent, preferring privacy as they explored their sexuality. "I preferred to go about it myself without telling her . . . she'd leave little things on my dresser about AIDS and safe sex. And she was concerned about it. But she left my private life private, which was good" (Joanna). Ann thought her mother "would have loved it if we had these great talks but I wasn't into that." Only Marianna's parents talked about sex before adolescence. Even though Donald's mother was an epidemiologist researching cervical cancer, the importance of using condoms was the extent of sex education on her part. Donald learned about sex from his stepfather's *Penthouse* magazines.

Shawn felt that his mother handled his sexuality in a positive way, one involving little discussion:

> A very smart thing that she did that I will do with my children forever, I mean, is that at the point where she started to sense that we were really getting sexually involved, she used to put condoms in our bathroom and ask no questions. Smartest thing she could ever do. Because it was . . . I think a lot of kids are embarrassed for some reason at, you know, age—how old, 15 or 16?—to walk in the supermarket and buy a box of condoms. I mean, it should also be like a law, that if you do go into a market, you know, for the person who's selling the condoms not to just, not to hassle that person at all, you know, because that is so, I mean I, I know, one of my brothers, like younger, or one of my friend's younger brother, he went into a market and he stole, he got caught shoplifting condoms, and it's just it's horrible to get caught, but I mean I think that that's a very good thing on the parents' part. You know, because children are gonna be stupid, teenagers especially.

Shawn felt that his mother gave him good advice (i.e., "just watch yourself,") but he felt that she was very open and honest, not judging him, but asking, "Shawn, are you sure about this?"

Rick's father told him to "be careful,"

> "Think before you act," he always said. And I think he puts the burden on me like he knows . . . he's entrusting me to be under control and everything so don't let him down, you know. So when I—if I decide to drink or if I decide to smoke a little bit tonight, don't, you know,

don't ruin the trust that he has in you. You know so it's like I'm doing it for me but more for him, because he, you know. . . . And for some reason it just works *so* good. It's like the way he looks at me or something is like, oh. . . . I can't, I'm gonna, I'm driving tonight, okay? You know, it's like I'm not doin' *anything* tonight, and. . . But he always says that, you know, always wear a condom.

After his first sexual experience, Rick's father asked him if he'd "used something."

Karen's mother took her to the doctor to get oral contraceptives but never did talk about sexuality. Mary's mother gave her "a technical explanation, like the penis goes to the vagina, it was 5 minutes long, and then I was like oh, okay, by that time I already knew. I just wanted to see what she was gonna tell me." When Leo asked his mother about sex,

> she freaked out. The next day after school she had a couple of books, *Where Do Babies Come From?* She just let us read them and she's all, "Any questions?" and we're too embarrassed and so we said no, my sister and I.

When he was "about 13, 14 my younger brother and I, [my stepfather] started talking about something about masturbation and something like that, 'oh, I bet you guys are doing it.' I think that's about the extent, the only time he mentioned sex with us." When Susannah's mother gave her a book, Susannah's reaction

> was like, "Psht. This is hokey." And then, later on, I think when I had my period she sat down and talked to me more about what happens when you have your period and all this stuff that, that as she was explaining it I'm like, "Yeah, whatever, I don't understand this stuff. Sure, okay." And then so she's like, "If you have any questions." And I think at that point if she had, if she would have talked to me later on again then it probably would have been better.

Like Karen's mother, Susannah's mother obtained birth control pills for her. Sonia's mother merely told her, " 'make sure they're not going out with you just for one thing because that's all guys want.' That's all she would say." Charlie's parents simply told him not to go out with girls until college. Before he left for Berkeley, his mother said,

> "All right, so I'll tell you one thing." I said, "What?" "Always wear a rubber." And I started laughing so hard and I actually said, "What!"

My dad said, "I don't know a thing. Don't ask me anything. I don't know anything that's going on." And my mom said, "No, really. Really. It's really dangerous out there. You should be really safe." And that's it, that's the only thing they ever told me. They never really told me anything else. I guess they always figured I'd find out myself, I don't know, from TV, from school.

DL: So when you were going through puberty they never explained any-thing?

Charlie: No, they never told us anything.

Although none of the participants had had extensive sex educa-tion at home, Charlie's family typified the experience of the Asians in the study. This was the only topic in which ethnicity emerged as an issue: Though many of the Asian students considered their par-ents more liberal than other Asian parents, they all described a phe-nomenon I called *active denial*, where their parents let them know they did not want to know about their childrens' romantic lives, even if it meant lying. As Vicky says,

They know like, they know I go out with guys 'cause they call obvi-ously, but I guess this is really, the culture does come in, huh? Um, I think that Chinese people are very into not necessarily lying but white lies. They would rather you believe something else and . . . I don't know what it is, but they would rather lie about how they're feeling and have you think they feel fine if you know we're at this social family occasion and my mom is having cramps per se, I mean, this is hypo-thetically speaking, and she'll act like nothing's wrong but she'll be suffering so much inside but because she's at this occasion and she can't leave because that would give "bad face"—I don't know, she'll sit there and be tormented through this whole thing but that's the Chinese way, I guess.

Vicky described how the phenomenon would be enacted in her family vis-à-vis dating:

I had my boyfriend over and he had his shoes at the front door and we weren't even doing it, we were like just in the back room watching TV and my parents came home. We heard the garage door open and I'm like, oh shit, you know, *get out of the house*. And they were coming upstairs and as they were coming upstairs, he grabbed his shoes and he ran outside so he's holding his shoes, running outside. My mom, for some reason, went outside. I don't know—I guess she dropped something outside when they were driving in so she walks outside and she sees this boy running up the street with his shoes in his hands, right, so I got kind of got in trouble for that but I mean, they know, like they'll catch me every so often but I lie to them. I mean I play it off because it's the only way that they'll be happy because that's their way of living, um, that they'd rather have me say, I'm going to the library and on a Friday night, for me to go clubbing. Sometimes I even take stuff to go change at my friend's house. It's gotten that bad.

Vicky thought her mother had found condoms in her purse while cleaning Vicky's room, but her mother wouldn't say anything. Vicky felt,

It's scary because I don't like her going through my stuff first of all. I don't like her knowing. See, it's gotten to the point where you don't even want her to know about your personal life, so, yeah it is bad. I mean you can't talk freely with her about it.

Charlie felt that he and his girlfriend couldn't be open about their relationship with their parents:

Charlie: Yeah. They, once in a while they ask her, like once in a while. Like every 4 or 5 months they'll ask her questions like what's my relationship with her, you know, like what does she think of me? But that's it. They don't want to, you know, they don't want to believe, they kind of look the other way.

DL: And what does she say when they ask her that?

Charlie: I think her answer was she "thinks well of me." It's in Chinese so it's like a rough translation, but it just meant like the translation is that she thinks well of me. So her parents basically know what that means, but they don't want to invade it, you know? Like they'll joke around with their, with their friends, like say that yeah that she has a guy that she hangs out with a lot. But they don't necessarily come out and say I'm her boyfriend. You know, they don't want to say it, like you know, my parents do the same thing. They don't, they don't really want to say it, they know it, you know, if it's gonna be anybody it's gonna be her, and it probably is her, but they don't want to say. I mean they ask, my mom asks me questions, like um, "Did you kiss her good-bye?" And I ask her "What?" And she goes all, "Nothing, nothing." And you know, they don't, they just don't want to see it.

Even though Ginger's mother asked direct questions, Ginger felt her mother didn't really want answers:

Ginger: Well my mom . . . she's like, "Why?" But she—I mean, she knows. I might even ask a question just completely just out of the blue, right? And everything sort of comes from you. And so, so she's like, "Why?" Um . . . "You're not . . . ?" And see, she can't even say the word.

DL: So she asked you directly?

Ginger: She asked me directly! I said, "No." And I think she asked me if I were gay, then that's in I'm sort of I guess being a politician about this—I'm like "No, I'm not *gay*." And um . . . And then she's . . . And I, I will ask in friends and in L.A., I mean that I met here, and she, she's . . . who lives really close to me and when we go to clubs and stuff and then my mom . . . Like for some reason asked me, "So are you guys dating?"

DL: She *asked* you?

Ginger: No she didn't—Yeah. She's like, "Is there something you want to tell me?" Like one time I came home, it was like around two and

DL: Sounds like she's open to hearing, if she would ask.

Ginger: No, she's not. . . . If they ask you, "Are you having sex?" they expect to hear a no. I mean it's like, they can't even . . . You know, "*Lie* to me, *please!*" You know? And you can see that in their eyes. So how can I tell them? Um, "Is there something going on?" and "Honestly. There isn't anything going on. Absolutely no."

The experience of these young people illustrates how discussing sex with adolescents in a superficial fashion without having previously established it as a legitimate topic of conversation prevents parents from being able to help prepare them for adult life in this important domain. Perhaps training parents to be more open and comfortable and to begin talking about sex at younger ages is less suitable than finding someone else to do a good job. In many cultures, it is the aunt or uncle or some other family member who is more removed, protecting the psychodynamics of the parent-child relationship. Parents may not be the appropriate people to be instructing their children about sex. Given the lack of extended family support for most Americans, one might expect the school to be a more fitting arena for sexual education than the home.

SEX EDUCATION IN THE UNITED STATES

Sex education in the public schools has been restricted by confusion over what knowledge is appropriate, yet discussion about sex in the United States has been surrounded by images of danger and victimization. Girls are taught to defend themselves against disease, pregnancy, and being "used" (Fine, 1988). Sexuality is presented variously as a biological function with little more symbolic meaning than elimination or as fundamentally coercive and violent. The range and diversity of sexuality is officially marked by silence. Sometimes, it is even actively censured, as in the case of the New York superintendent of schools who lost his job over New York's proposed Rainbow Curriculum, which was to be multicultural and sensitive to various sexual orientations. In religious terms, sex is taught as a moral value, temptation to be resisted and overcome. An image of sexuality as a positive, voluntary expression of desire or emotional commitment is largely missing from both school-based sex education and health policy discourse (Ehrhardt, 1996; Fine, 1988).

American parents generally believe that sex education should begin at home, taught by parents, though we have just seen that it doesn't happen. Over 80% of Americans also believe that sex education should be taught in school—only 2% to 7% of parents ask to have their children excused from sex education classes (Fine, 1988); however, there is controversy about what should be included in such curricula. Education programs are expected to stress abstinence in spite of the fact the average age of sexual debut is around 16 years. Some adults, represented by William Bennett, former federal Secretary of Education under George Bush, would have abstinence emphasized, teaching restraint and promoting sex only within the context of marriage. Others, notably the former Surgeons General C. Everett Koop and Jocelyn Elders, prefer to acknowledge the reality of teenage sexual activity, recommending the teaching of safer sex guidelines, assertiveness, and sexual negotiation skills, a stance that cost Dr. Elders her job. There has been no consensus in the United States about the most effective way to prepare young people for sexual activity and protect them against sexually related risks.

According to participants, school sex education must change before it can fulfill an education function abdicated by parents. As it was, school wasn't much more effective than parents for informing these students about sexuality. Sex was covered variously in health, family life, and safety classes. Most of these covered little more than the biology of human sexuality, without addressing the complexities of relationships. Few discussed STDs, and none the positive aspects of sex. Most participants were scarcely aware of HIV before they arrived at Berkeley. Whatever they included, sex education classes in high school had made very little impact.

Five men, George, Charlie, Sebastian, Donald, and Jacob, said that sex education in their schools had covered mainly what they all called the "mechanics." Rita, Janice, Joanna, Lauren, and Denise went to Catholic schools. Among them, only Janice thought her sex education had been adequate because it was given during all 4 years of high school, and the nuns had talked about different contraceptive methods; however, the abortion class had featured pictures of "chopped up fetuses." Sarita remembered sex education as being given early on in high school, but "no one really listened to what was going on. It was something that everyone was uncomfortable about and giggled about. And no one really absorbed all the information— and it wasn't relevant, either." Lauren offered a sole dissenting experience: Her class in the first year of high school taught about "protection, they taught about what sex is, different kinds of sex, and about being gay, being straight, being whatever. And that was a really good class, and that had me knowing it." Sebastian, Jacob, and Dave were bothered about the lack of information about homosexuality: Dave found it difficult not having role models in high school, even thinking of suicide after his first sexual encounter. Sebastian didn't find the anonymous question box in his class useful because he was too intimidated to ask his questions, but Hanan thought the one in her class had been helpful.

Hanan and Andrew were the only students who learned about AIDS and the use of condoms with spermicide during high school. Susannah, Ann, and Sonia didn't remember what they'd learned about sex in school. Ann's attitude about the assemblies during AIDS Awareness week was, "You'd hear the same thing year after year after year, until you were like 'Can I just get up there and say it myself? Can I test out of assembly today?' " She didn't feel that high school sex education had had much of an impact on her: "It wasn't effective because it wouldn't change anyone's behavior." George thought sex education classes should emphasize the psychosocial through the use of role-playing. Susannah had recently done a paper on the family life education class at Berkeley High, and admired the amount of attention they spent on self-esteem, confidence, and treating others respectfully, "trying to get students to feel good about themselves so they didn't feel like they needed to go out and have sex." She took a summer course on sexuality at UC Berkeley that she thought was thorough and useful.

Several others mentioned how helpful the health education class from which I recruited them had been. Vicky felt that because of the class, she was able to negotiate openly in a sexual situation with another member of the class, where someone who hadn't taken the class wouldn't have understood. Charlie and Sonia had begun using spermicidal foam as a result of the class, Joanna felt she'd become more tolerant and accepting of diversity, and Theresa felt that students in her section had been enlightened in a positive way.

Friends

Normative pressure among friends occurs not just with respect to sexual behavior; it refers to a constellation of social behaviors that also include drinking and smoking. How and whether friends liked talking about sex and practiced safer sex were strong influences in predicting whether a participant was having safer sex. People often seek friends with similar values, which they reinforce for each other. When friends don't practice safer sex, it becomes more difficult to imagine doing so. In cases where an individual's values are dissonant with the friends', a tension exists where they may try to influence each other or where one of them is independently trying to incorporate the values of the friends.

These processes and influences are not necessarily conscious: George, a health education tutorial leader, compared his sexual behavior to his smoking, and although he recognized that he and his peers shared behaviors, he denied that the milieu could have any normative influence on either behavior.

> See, I'm slowly incorporating a lot of those ideas into a behavioral change in myself. You know, I smoke, and I teach about tobacco use and how bad it is, but I smoke. My mom smokes and she's a nurse. So, I think that in overcoming personal change, like for myself, you have to take yourself out of the situation, you have to look at why you smoke, and you have to take yourself out of the situations. One of the reasons I smoke is because 10 other guys in the house smoke and I'm constantly around them, and I live here. . . . Yeah, it's not peer pressure to smoke. What I said is, is I live in a house where people smoke. It's different, it's different. . . . Peer pressure is having someone say, oh, do you know how bad smoking is for you, or why don't you just smoke, come on, everybody's doing it type of thing. But when you're in a house where a lot of people smoke, you're around that environment and it's not peer pressure, it's the availability, it's being able to oh easily go upstairs and do, I know this person smokes maybe I'll go ask him for a cigarette, maybe I'll go and have a conversation with him after lunch and we'll have a cigarette, so it's not, it's different, there's no peer pressure involved.

Hanan, Lauren, Jacob, Sonia, and Charlie were especially concerned with encouraging their friends. Hanan felt that she and her dorm-mates had been "one big happy family, all these brothers and three little sisters," and as such were entitled to give each other advice. She discouraged smoking and made certain that when floormates got drunk, they wore unconstricting clothing for when they passed out and had wastebaskets nearby in case they vomited. She felt strongly about encouraging friends to bring condoms along in any dating situation. Dave, too, offered his friends condoms on their way out. Lauren and her friends monitored each others' behaviors: "The first one says, 'Did you guys have sex?' 'Yeah.' 'Did you use protection?' And that's the rule. We just ask each other." Rick told his friend about a new partner,

> and the first thing I was telling it to him and he's just like, "Well you used something, right?" And I'll be like, "Yeah, I did." We're so close knit, it's like that's the first thing. We always take care of each other. And it's really weird, 'cause it's, for me, and our friends, it's like a given.

Jacob was known to his friends as "Joe Safe Sex." His attitude was, "if it's available, why not use it?" His friends felt they could call on him, to the extent that he'd driven condoms and lubricant over to a friend in the middle of the night. "A lot of my friends say, 'Geez, I wished everyone practiced safer sex like you do.' And they even say that they wish they did too." After an unplanned pregnancy, Sonia felt it her "mission" to make sure her brothers and sisters were protected and even offered to obtain condoms for them. Charlie felt that his friends could be divided between those who'd had sex and the ones who hadn't. Those who had would give useful advice, but the others would just joke around without being able to offer anything substantive. Talking about sex was a way of giving and receiving support as well as providing a normative influence and did not necessarily have to be about safe sex to set the climate. It was a way of taking care and showing each other that care.

GENDER DIFFERENCES IN SEX TALK AMONG FRIENDS

The manner in which talk about sex occurred varied by gender, for both men and women felt they could speak more openly with women. Five participants mentioned that joking was a way for men to cloak their vulnerability, ignorance, or embarrassment to communicate about sex. The contrast in gender was significant: where

Lauren and her flatmates discussed relationships, they were very frank with each other, enabling a forum for the normative influence demonstrated earlier:

> We're really open about, me and my friends are really open about it. We break it down to each other. I was telling Mark that, I said, "Yeah," I said, "I know how you do it, what you do, what you look like," and he says "No-o." I said, "Don't be—" I said, "I can break it down," I said, "You don't know how much girls talk."

Charlie and his friends felt the same freedom to be open with each other, particularly concerning sexual experience:

> No, because if you play it as if you do, right, when something really happens or some real question comes up, you have to come out and say, well, I've never really had sex. And that, that's even more embarrassing to have to admit it, when it counts the most, rather than someone just asking you—I think. Or that's what we think, actually, all of us. That's why, well, my friends who don't have sex, they always answer "no" right away. And my friends who have sex, we, we have all these joking answers. Say, "Well, I don't know if it's good enough to call it *sex*," but, or whatever, I don't know. It's better than sex, I wouldn't call it sex. I don't know. We joke around. We never give a straight answer.

Charlie and Andrew impressed me with the depth of their feelings for their girlfriends, but Charlie explained how they weren't permitted to express it.

> Um, there's uh just the plain physical level. That's the level of saying yeah, you could describe like some of the things that happened and you could describe like how good it was or uh how many times you did it or you know, or what she was doing while you were doing it, what she was saying or stuff like that. But you never, we never go down to the level to say you know, how much it means to you, right, how it affects you if like you're making love to one girl then the next day she like treats you like crap. And you know, we never really talk about that.

Joseph felt that men had fewer ways to express their feelings about relationships than women, "as far as defining them." He explained the semantics of the gender difference:

> Usually, guys won't say, "I made love to this girl," unless they really, really care for that girl. Um . . . They just say, "yeah, I fucked her," or

"we've slept together" or "we've done it." Whereas with girls, it depends what kind of relationship you have with the girls, the guys kind
of, it's all the same with guys, you know, as far as what you would
use. You would only use, you would only say you made love to this
girl to a close friend, whereas with regular friends, with other guys,
you'd just say you slept with her. And if you're talking to a girl, I don't
think you would say "I fucked her," say, you know, to your friend,
well, "we slept together." I think you would say different things.

Joseph explained the function of joking among men as "a way they
kind of protect themselves, they say it, and they express their feelings, but just in case there's someone who would make a joke out of
it, they can go along with it, I think." Andrew and his friends needed
to start talk about sex in a joking way but could sometimes progress
to more serious conversation,

> Actually my friends, my friends and I, I mean one of the reasons I
> choose them is 'cause they, they are okay with that sometimes. I think
> my friends are okay with it, they can joke, but at the same time, the
> conversation will settle down and they will talk about it seriously. We
> will talk about it seriously. And I think, I have friends who just like
> you know, you know you'll start talking to them seriously and they'll
> be like, "Oh, c'mon, man." And they'll go back to the joking. But, and
> I think one of the reasons I like the people that I stay talking with about
> those things is because they can sit down and know when to be serious.

Eric told me that as he and his roommate were getting to know
each other, each felt it necessary to exaggerate the extent of his sexual
experience, "but then as we started to know each other and feel comfortable around each other, the truth started coming out from both of
us." He felt that "all guys are like that," but learning to be more
truthful with Uri had allowed him the freedom not to lie with fellow
football players in the locker room. A few men had noticed the difference in the extent and quality of conversation possible with their
male and their female friends. Rick felt he needed to joke with male
friends—"we'll be joking and just say the most disgusting perverted
things," but "then when we want to, we can get down serious and a
lot of girls come to me and my friends just to talk." Leo, who was gay,
talked to male friends about sex, but "with my two close straight
female friends, yeah, I tell them what I do, and they're very explicit."
Joseph commented that

> there's certain girls that you can strike up these types of conversations
> with and there's others that you know that they don't feel comfortable

with it, so you use different words. You get the same information, just in a different way.

Andrew now trusted a couple of his male friends but had formerly only talked to women.

It's funny, it used to be that I could only talk about it to women. I had a little trouble talking about it with men and I was just, I remember one of my professors saying how sad it was that men didn't talk to other men about their sex lives enough. So I think it's also maturation.

He and Jacob presented attitudes that offered hope for the future. Jacob summed up the importance of talking about sex with friends,

I guess our philosophy is, "Hey it's the nineties." In this day and age, you can't just go "Hush. Hush. Hush." And besides, we have no reason to feel embarrassed about it at all. Just like I don't feel embarrassed going into a drugstore or supermarket and buying condoms. I'll put them there with my groceries. I couldn't care less what people think about me.

THE INFLUENCE OF FRIENDS' BEHAVIOR

Besides the overt influence in how friends talk about sex with each other, their personal behavior affords a subtle influence in the ability to imagine safer sex. Janice felt frustrated because she considered herself a strong feminist, yet she was unable to get her boyfriend to use condoms. Her friends had similar problems, and they all found refusing sex difficult with their partners, "they had to because if they didn't give it to him, he could get it from somewhere else. That's what sort of made their relationship unique was that they got sex from this person and not any other person." In spite of their feminism, they weren't able to model assertive behavior for each other, making alternatives difficult to envision. Similarly, Ann didn't know anyone practicing safer sex and couldn't imagine that any of her peers were. Most of Ann's friends were on the pill, "most of the people I think I've ever known. I mean, ever since I—back to high school or something, and it's just something everybody did."

DL: Do you have any friends who are "doing all the right things," as you say?

Ann: Uh, I don't know if anybody really does in that even, even when you think you're safe, it's like I said, a lot of my friends that—and

myself included—that have their boyfriends have decided we're
safe, so as long as we stay together we're safe. It's like trying to build
a little island or something where no one can get at you. So I, I don't
know if that's right because—then again, how do you really know?

DL: But do you have any friends who have said, "If a guy comes near me
without a condom, I'm not doing it."

Ann: No. No.

The people Raphael knew at school had influenced his attitudes
about using condoms for fellatio. Even though he thought "it would
be kind of fun, almost" to practice "*safer* safer sex," he didn't because
he felt "that other people don't want to use them" because,

> most people that I've talked to about it don't like the taste of condoms
> or anything. Or don't like to bother with them. So I guess that's why
> I feel like they don't . . . I've heard friends talking about it, or I'm sure
> I've been in the conversation too, in saying, you don't like the taste of
> condoms or something like that.

His closest friends were all elsewhere, and these he thought were
"more safe than I am, I'd say."

Among athletes, Eric informed me, there was no particular pressure to engage in safer sex; indeed, there was some pressure against
using condoms by teasing those who helped themselves to the condoms supplied in the locker room in an upturned helmet. "The only
comments that'll be made are 'Why are you taking those? You won't
be needing those.' That's the only comment I've ever heard, not 'You
shouldn't be doing that,' or stuff like that. Nothing like that." I in-
quired, "So if a guy would say 'I was with this girl last weekend and
I'm with another girl this weekend,' nobody will say 'Aren't you
worried about that?' "No" he said, "Nothing like that."

George's attitudes had been shaped by his brother and a close
friend. Though the brother and friend had both contracted STDs,
because they had been easily resolved, George had no fear of STDs.
Friends are therefore an important source of information and support, influencing each other in both positive and negative ways. They
encourage or inhibit safer sex behavior and attend to each other during periods of experimentation.

Student Life and Drinking

Alcohol is the wheel that makes social life at university revolve,
especially during the first year. Although people went to bars to drink

and socialize, parties seemed to be focal in the social process. Whereas parties occurred at people's houses, fraternities were mentioned as the most usual site for first-year students to experience their newfound freedom.

PARTYING FIRST YEAR

Whether or not it was associated with a fraternity, the first semester or year at university was a time to explore through partying, drinking, and sex. Drinking and sex were both expressions of freedom; one was not contingent on the other. Although people did engage in sexual exploration because of drinking, they also drank to allow themselves the freedom to experiment. Sarita had had a sheltered upbringing and enjoyed the freedom of being away from home:

> I thought, yeah I definitely do want to lose my virginity. And I thought about it and I wanted to just go out there and date and do all the things that I couldn't do before. . . . So I went to a lot of parties and I guess the aim of a lot of those parties is get drunk and get together with somebody.

Her roommate

> became sexually active with some people that the next morning she didn't remember what had happened and we had to tell her "oh, you went with that guy." I mean I don't know exactly what occurred, because she willingly went wherever. The guys had their rooms there, so she would go. She would leave and I know a couple times as she was leaving, I'd say, "Do you know what you're doing, are you sure you want to go?" She's like "yeahyeahyeah. I want to go." So I guess in that sense, I guess by going upstairs with someone you pretty much consent.

Denise felt that she had consented:

> When I first got into the sorority, there's tons of drinking and I guess the two times that I slept with two people because I was completely, I think that was my first 2 weeks in the house, I was completely drunk I didn't even, and I had never drank in high school, I went and I went in to the sorority and we had a pledge event and they were giving us upside-down margaritas and um it's like when they bend you over and they pour tequila and drinks down your throat and if you didn't do it I mean I guess peer pressure but you felt like kind of stupid because everyone else was doing it and all the guys are around there so if you and all your pledge sisters are doing it and you don't you're

like well . . . and you're a freshman and you're already confused as it is it just seems like, fine I'll just do it. And, um, that's when I actually had like just random sex. I don't even know if it was protected, you know it was that type of sex.

Andrew managed to maintain control sexually, but just barely.

Andrew: Yeah, but I remember going to the couch, *foom*, last person at the party kind of thing, fell asleep, and it was like, woke up and it was happening and I was, I remember going, okay, what do I do, and I was like, "Hey, wait, nonononono."

DL: Did you feel offended or violated?

Andrew: Her and I used to go out, you know, and I—

DL: But you still hadn't given your consent.

Andrew: Exactly, exactly, yeah, but I was kind of but—you know when you're drunk, I could have been asleep, I could have been maybe, I'd never blacked out before. Ever. But I felt, I remember going and closing my eyes and dreaming and maybe I could have been awake or said something to her, or made some kind of motion or something. When you are drunk you never know, so I wasn't exactly in a position, 'cause I wasn't sure about what had happened, what I had said or had done before that, even though I was laying. So I wasn't in the position to say, "Hey, what the hell are you doing?"

Jacob had a period where he never went out without getting drunk first and where he would get into fights and have to be taken home by his friends. There were several evenings he didn't remember. Nonetheless, he felt certain he had not had unsafe sex. He said,

I feel confident that no matter how altered my senses are, I think I would still do some things the same. I mean, I've had dreams and in my dreams I have, *I have safer sex*. I mean in my dreams and I'll even know that I'm dreaming about this and still I will have safer sex.

Rick's experience didn't involve unremembered sex, but was also typical.

That—the first semester I didn't play [football], I like just came out this semester so um the first semester I was just slacking, goofing off, you know, drinking with the guys in the room, not do—"Ah, homework— I'll do it tomorrow," you know, and it was just not good. And I was just enjoying being in college, I think. . . . That was bad, that was bad.

Like in the first 2 weeks—we took pictures, too, 'cause my roommate, Dean, we went to high school together and we decided to room together. And the two other roommates we had, we got along with really good and dadada, and it was just, we just clicked and it was just a lot of fun to just be around 'em, so . . . And so we're living on our own and everything, and it was cool. And um the first 2 weeks I think we took pictures of when we brought home the beer. We went through 11 or 12 cases of beer. We just, we just—drinking, just during the week, we were just like, "oh my god," you know, just . . . And then like after that we looked at the pictures of ourselves, 'cause we took pictures with all the beer boxes, you know, the 12-packs, and we were just like, "What were we thinking?" You know, in the middle of the semester— like *fuck* you know? What the hell were we thinking, you know, and what are we here for?

After this initial period, most students put their partying into perspective and settled down a bit, but partying during the first or second semester seemed to fill an important need to express newfound freedom away from parents and community of origin.

MEN AND DRINKING

Although both men and women liked to drink, the pressure to get drunk was stronger for men. Drinking was used to help men share their feelings, creating an atmosphere in which bonding could occur. Rita speculated on the difference in pressure when I asked her whether her role as a nondrinking sorority president had any normative influence on the other members in her house:

No. [laughs] Definitely not. Mmm, I think in all the houses, there are people who don't drink, who don't drink at all just because of either religious or just personal preference or things like that. Even in fraternities, there are guys who don't drink. And I think that when they—I think the peer pressure comes in when it's the guys who always boast that they drink a lot, or, they're like, oh yeah, you know, I can down this six-pack in 5 seconds, or something like that. It's those guys who get the peer pressure more because they're boasting about it to drink more. Peer pressure to drink basically when they don't want to drink because they're always saying, yeah, I can drink. So that when they're out at a social event where there's drinking, people expect them to. I think that's more the peer pressure, at least what I've seen. Compared to the people who at the start say, I don't drink so that's just the way I am. People don't pressure those people to drink. So—because I have seen guys who don't drink at fraternities. And are popular. I mean, supposedly in the popular fraternities, there are those guys who don't drink. And they're very popular guys. I really think it's how you present yourself in the beginning when you join the house, or when you first meet people, and when you say "I don't drink" in the beginning, people do respect that. But if you're a person who's kind of wavering and doesn't really have a definite answer, and wants to be the cool guy and try to follow . . . follow everyone's lead, those are the people who get in trouble from what I've seen.

DL: A lot of people do experimenting when they first get to—

Rita: Yeah, that's true too. I know I did, because the high school I went to was very different compared to other people. Just because we didn't have, or at least I wasn't in a group where we had parties and drank and did all that stuff. And my friends and I, we would go out and we'd do different things to have fun. Like go to the beach and ya know and get a beach pit, and goof off, and have beach fires. We never really drank or stuff like that. So I never really had that peer pressure to drink and I never drank 'til I came to college. So I definitely experimented with alcohol my first semester here.

Rick speculated on the norms that encourage men to drink. First, there was the use of alcohol to facilitate expressiveness between men:

I mean, there's times where we just kick back or even sometimes when we just have, we just feel like one, I mean, and we'll just sit back and we'll start talking. 'Cause we get really deep conversations, like last night we talked about 2 hours about religion and stuff, it was just, it was kind of cool. And we were sittin' there drinkin', you know, just drank one beer and just . . . You know, maybe it's a bonding, male bonding thing you have to have a beer in your hand or something, I don't know, but . . .

Yet in groups, getting drunk or holding one's alcohol was considered a feat that facilitated the bonding.

Rick: Yeah. I think it's just because . . . it's just something that you have to, you know, that little high school adolescent or you know, drinking in college attitude where you gotta be able to uh say, "oh yeah, I was really drunk that night," and "oh I did this many shots and I drank this much." It's like a, like a you know competition or something, to see who's been drunk more times or something, or . . . It's just something that you don't perceive as fun or not in your own mind because it's something you're doing for the value of storytelling type thing.

DL: So it's like a rite of passage.

Rick: Yeah. Exactly.

DL: Is it the same for guys and girls? Are the standards the same, do you think?

Rick: I'm not sure, I really couldn't say, but from what I've . . . from what I see, my opinion, I think . . . I think guys, sometimes it gets to be more of like a macho thing, like, "oh, I drank a 12-pack by myself in an hour," you know? And or I bonged this many beers in like 10 minutes, or I did this many shots. I think that's—if anything, that's what the guy thing and the mentality is. It's like a macho thing. But for girls I don't, I really couldn't say. I think . . . I'm not sure, because it's a lot easier for girls not to drink. I don't know why.

DL: There's less pressure?

Rick: Yeah. Maybe. And that's because, just simply because it's the guy thing, it's like a macho thing. "You not drinkin', how come you're not drinking? You got a beer in your hand there," you know, something like that. But girls, I don't think it's really like a big deal. I don't know if it is or isn't. There's some that do drink a lot, there's some that don't.

Several students commented on athletes and their reputations. Athletes were known to attend class less often, partly because they were often excused for athletic practice or games. For this reason perhaps, only two participants were members of sports teams. Eric felt that he and his roommate were at Berkeley to get their degrees, but the other athletes acted as though they were there "to play football and maybe I'll go to class once in a while." He felt that their attitudes reflected on him, and it disappointed him when they "walk in late with a strut—they have the hugest egos." George, Denise, and Hanan spontaneously mentioned the homophobia of athletes. Denise added that

> the ones that are homophobic seem to be pretty open about it and they'll do it in groups. Maybe 'cause it strengthens their community, it's really easy to attack someone when you're with your friends and they feel stronger when they do that.

According to Denise, in preparation for the health education class in which a gay-lesbian-bisexual panel was planned, the instructor felt it necessary to separate the athletes and fraternity members to temper the homophobic remarks that would result from group encouragement. Even George commented on the homophobia of the athletes in his tutorial group, at the same time coming across as a stereotypically homophobic fraternity member.

FRATERNITIES, STUDENT LIFE, AND DRINKING

Fraternity parties came up as an important center of student life, particularly during a student's first year; several people mentioned the "Thursday night parties." Although one could theoretically go to a fraternity party and not drink, drinking and perhaps meeting a potential partner were perceived as the point of the parties. George reflected on the casual and unsafe sexual behavior he observed:

> You just meet them and having sex with them and not communicating about things. I mean it happens, it happens. I don't want to say it happens here a lot, because then I would be saying it happens to fraternity guys. It happens on this campus a lot.

George was aware of the stereotypes about fraternity members and the stigma associated with them:

> I think the image of fraternities is really distorted I think. This house, like I said before, is really diverse. We have people who sleep with a lot of women, we have people who sleep with some women, we have some that don't sleep with women at all. We're not all alcoholics.

Yet George's attitudes fit my idea of quintessential fraternity behaviors and attitudes, and several of the women's experiences corresponded with this view.

> Janice: But then again, the three guys who are in the class are the fraternity type. To me that means that they had to have had women by now. That's part of their initiation into a fraternity, and that's what they do on their Thursday night parties. I have a sort of negative viewpoint of fraternity men but that's . . . I know when I first came here, a couple of the guys I messed around with, that's all you could call it, were fraternity guys. They just wanted women and that was that. They didn't want relationships. They didn't want . . . even though they acted like it. I remember this one guy. I was sitting on his dorm bed with him, actually, laying in it with him, and he was telling me this story. His brother drowned and he was, like, making moves on me while he was telling me this. I laughed because I thought he was joking. And he said, "How can you laugh when I'm telling you this

deep emotional story about myself?" But you've got your hand in my robe, what do you mean? So that struck me as funny that they were mixing this deep emotion with sex. And I thought that was a total joke.

Rita thought that "this whole fraternity scene in my freshman year had a lot to do with a lot of people were not remembering what they had done and waking up with diseases and just not knowing what had happened." Rita had had a similar experience during her first year.

> I forgot about this one guy, this one guy that I went out with actually. Because I didn't really have that experience of dating guys and stuff like that. So this one guy, the first date, he was a fraternity guy. He asked me, "Oh, do you wanna go back and hang out for awhile?" And I assumed it was hang out with everybody else. But it wasn't what he was talking about . . . So we went back to his house and he brought me in the back way and we ended up going to his room. And he was like, "Oh, this is my room," and he had a single, which was very convenient for him. And I was like, "Oh great, what is he thinking?" Then he started kissing me and um after a while, he started doing some other stuff and everything and I said, "I'm really not comfortable with this." He said, "Why not?" I'm just, "I'm not. This is my first date with you. I don't know you well enough to go through with, to go all the way." He's like, "Why? Everyone does it. I don't understand." He like really reminded me of the typical fraternity guy that people talk about, where these guys just take these girls out just to have sex sort of thing, he really reminded me of that. He really pushed me pretty much to my limits. But I finally just said no and basically just walked out of there and never talked to him again.

Rita wasn't much of a drinker so was able to refuse the man's advances and have him take her seriously. In drinking situations, women weren't always as clear thinking or assertive.

Rick and his friend were against fraternities at first. They went out to the recruiting events for the free food, but ended up pledging. He explained their metamorphosis—note the transition from "they" to "we:"

> The guys—see, when I—when uh we started rushing the week that you can go look around all the other houses. Shane and I were just like, you know, they give really good meals there, so we were just going around just eating like ribs here, steak and lobster here, and we were just like, you know, "This is great!" and uh and we're just totally against it. It's the stereotypical frats you know that just the frat guys

and it was just the Greek system is just not us. We don't need the social support, we can find our own friends, we don't need that. It's just so gay it's just so stereotypical BS. You know. And we're walking around and stuff and just went to a couple of houses, one house was all white and we're just all white guys and we're just like "What is this?" and then we went to one place and it was a total sales pitch. We walked in and the guys all, "How you doing, dudes? This is our house, let me show you around um this is where we have, this is where we usually are bars down there where the kegs are usually." And uh then take us upstairs to the balcony, and "this is a great place to take chicks and they can look out over the bay," and we're just like, we're going like, "Oh great" looking at each other like this is *exactly* what we just, you know, we're just laughing because it's just so dumb. And once we walked by this other house. This was just Sig Ep where I'm—we're at now. Um this—one of our other roommates, there was three of us at the time walking around, he knew somebody in that house and he said the guy said to stop by 'cause he wanted to talk to Ken our other roommate just 'cause he hadn't seen him in a while. So all right, so we stopped by and we walked in and we just did the whole schmiel—put our name tag on and you sign in and everything. Just to get some food you know and we walk in and uh all the brothers in the house are out there you know just introducing themselves they're just, you know, they just stand around. It was like a little social gathering or something. They were just—it was like, "Hey, how you doing?" you know, "My name is so and so" and they'd come up to you and say "Hi. My name is James," you know, "How are you doing?" and just, "Where are you from?" And the first night they didn't say anything about the house. They just asked how you were doing, you know. Yeah, and they seemed sincere about it, too. Not just like trying to get you to be in their house because we need a quota to fill or something you know. But um they, they were just, it was really sincere and it was just . . . And they found out about you rather than a sales pitch, "Come join our fraternity right away." They were all "let's get some food," you know it—"the guys're all here, let's get some food," you know. They just served it up and it was really cool. And then at the end of the night, we left and they were all, "Come back tomorrow night, at least for the food," you know and "See you again," or something. And we were just like, "Yeah, cool" you know, and we left and we're looking at each other and it was just we saw everybody. It was the only diverse house on this campus that we'd seen, Chinese, Mexicans, Blacks, Filipinos, what else was in there, you know just just a conglomeration of everything. I mean just, just a trip. It was like, that's what we want and they were—then the second night we went back, that's when we started asking about the house. We said, "Well, give us some input on the house," 'cause we were like considering it now, we were considering rushing now. We were like, "Oh god, what are we doing?" but we were still—at least we wanted to find out now because we could very likely fit into this house. And they were just stressing their academics as a priority, they've done sports because our house is really athletic, we like reign in the intramurals, right, and um, and then, you know, the community involvement, we try to do. So those are the three things that we try to stress and everything.

Denise's experience with community service while a sorority member was to "have a party for a certain project and there'll be beer and it'll be bring a fraternity over." Dave was invited to join a fraternity because he was a football player. Knowing he was "a major closet case back then," he declined. Hanan observed that when her dormmates joined fraternities, "their big change in life was drinking a lot." When I asked Sarita whether one could attend a fraternity party without drinking, she noted,

> Now, yes, but this was 4 years ago. I'm sure they could, but the main point of it was to go there and drink. I think with all my friends who are in the same year as I am in school, we basically outgrew them in one semester, or basically by the time it was our sophomore year, we didn't want to go any more. It wasn't fun.

Rita explained that "they didn't really have that many rules at the parties, so anyone could go, and you didn't have to be in that house either. So it was really easy to go to all these parties and not really have to deal with all the rules that the university and the international fraternities and sororities wanted us to have." George's fraternity had resisted the university limits on alcohol, with the support of their national group. During football season, his house would get *20 kegs* of beer for a weekend party. George explained his attitudes about drinking to me.

DL: How often are there parties here?

George: During the fall, during football season, every weekend. We have beer every weekend. Basically, we have beer pretty much on tap. If you go downstairs, we have a bar downstairs, where we have what's called a kegerator. Where you have beer on tap.

DL: I thought there were rules now.

George: There are. There's new rules, but it's—for me to explain it, it's a long story, but basically it's called the BYOB [bring your own bottle] policy, where you're not supposed to have kegs allowed in the house. Our national, now the reason that they're doing that is because there's 43 fraternities, 16 sororities on this campus. And people's national charters are starting to get pressure from insurance companies. In a case where there was a party and somebody got drunk from the beer that we supplied, and they went out and they got in a car accident and killed somebody, we could get sued. Now, our national, there's only two fraternities on this campus that have nationals that support kegs. Ours is one of them. This house and another house. That support kegs.

DL: Your national says it's okay?

George: Our national says it's okay. The IFC says it's not. The IFC, Inter-Fraternity Council here at Berkeley, says it's not. So, for big parties, like theme parties that we have, we have to incorporate the rules of the IFC.

DL: So, if it's an interfraternity . . .

George: If it's an interfraternity thing, but—

DL: If it's a house party?

George: If it's a house party, we can have alumni supply kegs. We're still not supposed to have house funds going towards kegs. I mean, it's just never—here, with the type of people you have, I don't think we're going to follow that. Especially now that we have, even though we have the new IFC vice president in this house, it's not gonna really make a difference because we think it's bullshit for the IFC to come in and say you guys can't have kegs. You know, we're our own organization. We decide our own rules. Co-ops decide their own rules. Why can't we?

DL: So there's no rules about co-ops having kegs?

George: I don't think so. Not to my knowledge. And the thing that upsets me so much, is how the Greek system gets incorporated into your alcoholics, your women-bashing, your men-bashing, your wild drunk people. When if you've ever been to a co-op and seen the way co-ops party, they not only abuse alcohol, but they abuse all kinds of drugs. Whether it's ecstasy, acid, marijuana, they're doing things right there.

DL: And that doesn't happen here?

George: Well, people abuse marijuana, but people don't abuse hard-core drugs like heroin, ecstasy—I don't know anybody in this house that has taken ecstasy, and so forth. But, I think that oftentimes the Greek systems here, and everywhere, gets put into this image where we're in the spotlight. We are supposed to be the role models, therefore, you cannot do anything that is harmful. You know, oh you can't drink, you're not supposed to have kegs, where they're not looking at the whole problem. The problem is university based. University, I mean, co-ops, dorms, there's alcoholics living in the dorms. There's alcoholics, there's drug users, you know, even in their own apartments. You've got to start—if you want to campaign, you can't start at the Greek system. You've got to start at the root of the problem. Which is why people socialize around alcohol. And why people socialize around drugs, and do educational workshops. But what the IFC is trying to do is, they're trying to get the easy way out, and they're just saying, okay we've adopted this BYOB policy that says you're not supposed to have kegs and if you have parties you can only bring six beers and you have to bring six beers to the party the day before, and you get issued little tickets. Which is not getting to the root of the problem. They're trying to curb drinking. You don't curb drinking by saying you can only drink six beers because what happens is the real alcoholics will preparty, and they'll go down the street, and they'll go to Henry's [a local pub] and they'll drink before they go to the party. You're not solving the problem. You're even helping it. You're telling people it's okay to go down the street and spend money on beer and stuff, then go to the party. And what you're doing is, you're going to get drunk people coming to the parties and then drinking more beer. Whereas before it's like, okay, let's leave for a party at 9:00, and you haven't had a beer yet, and you go to the party and you start drinking at maybe 9:00 or 10:00. But now, what's gonna happen, and it's happening already, is people go down the street, they go to bars, they get drunk, they buy their own beer, and maybe come up here and socialize around it here, and then go to the party. Which is just, for alcoholics, makes things so much worse.

DL: Do you have an idea how many people in this house are alcoholics? Or have alcohol problems?

George: About five.

DL: Out of 33?

George: About 33. Now, what I deem alcoholic might not be what you deem alcoholic. I think alcohol—if you're an alcoholic, abusing alcohol is one thing, see, I have a brother who's gotten two DUIs [traffic citations for driving under the influence of alcohol or drugs], okay. He's not an alcoholic. He has to go to programs because of the law that says, "You're an alcoholic." They make you seem like an alcoholic. He has made some bad choices. We talked about this this weekend. He's made some bad choices and he's probably abused alcohol, okay. It doesn't mean he's an alcoholic. To me, an alcoholic is when it starts coming into play habitually and you rely on it. Whether you get up in the morning and you drink, you act, you could talk like you and I are talking, and I'm drunk, and I still don't sound like I'm making sense. I don't go to my classes, I don't think that anything's important. You could just drink Friday and Saturday, or you could just drink on the weekend. And not be an alcoholic. Is *my* opinion of it. I think it's when it starts coming into play where it starts affecting your life so much that it reflects how your goals are. If I started drinking and I didn't do well in my classes and my long-term goal right now is to get through school and get a Bachelor's degree, move on. That's a goal right there. That's my first goal. Now if alcohol started, or drugs started coming to a point where I wasn't going to my classes, I was starting to get on AP [academic probation], these things were happening, then I would maybe start questioning that, yeah, I'm relying on alcohol. But I go out, and I drink every week, you know, I go out and I drink weekends, I go out with my friends, and I party, but look at the positions I hold: I'm a TA [teaching assistant], I'm in the band, I incorporate myself, I'm very politically active on this campus. You know. It's not affecting me to the point where it's taking control of my life. And that's—when you go to those AA [Alcoholics Anonymous] meetings, they don't get to the root of the problem. You get 30 people in a room and all of a sudden a guy goes up and he says, "Okay. The reason you guys are here is because you're all alcoholics." Which may or may not be the case.

George was right: what he considered alcoholic differed dramatically from my own definition; yet even from his own admittedly narrow definition, 15% of house members had problems with alcohol. His views on alcohol, peer pressure, and consent, combined with his general lack of awareness, were even more disturbing because he was a tutorial group leader with an open forum in which to have a weekly impact on student views.

This lengthy excerpt illustrates common attitudes about drinking on campus. Although partying is a part of university life that affects sexual behavior in important ways, parties are but one site for the genesis of sexual relationships. In the next section, I will describe ways in which relationships are formed and what these different types of relationships imply about how communication about sexuality can occur.

4

Negotiating Relationships

According to participants, relationships evolve as either casual or romantic, with partners beginning as strangers or friends, each form with its own implications for the construction of trust, communication, and how safe-sex issues are handled. Sexual negotiation is defined by impression management and bound by gender. This chapter outlines how sex is negotiated within different types of relationships.

Casual Relationships

The first type of liaison begins between strangers who have had no prior acquaintance. These are mainly casual dyads, which become sexual early on, before trust can be established. Such partners may have met serendipitously, at a party, a bar, a café, or book store. If they are short term or otherwise remain casual, risk can be assumed and appropriate precautions taken. If sex is used to create intimacy, that is, if a relationship beyond casual sex is intended, partners may talk about their previous relationships as a way of getting to know each other that signals their past risk behavior and investigates the other's. Neither the topic of safe sex nor the specific precautions one intends to take will have been discussed beforehand.

The second type of relationship begins with a date. Even though they were not previous acquaintances, one or both members of the couple may have noticed each other at work, school, or some other point on their normal trajectory. In this situation, they may use friends to gain information about a person or to disclose interest without risking rejection, as Eric did, "I noticed her one day and just told one of her friends and then she told her friends and it all got back to the big circle that you know, you should ask her out."

A potential partner's appearance is used to judge his or her safety more where the relationship begins between strangers than between acquaintances or friends. In the first condition of sexual friendship, the relationship has always been defined as that of nonromantic friends, although there may have been periods of sexual attraction. Particular conditions seem to be necessary for the relationship to turn sexual: Members of the pair must be attracted to each other at the same point in time (for often the attraction is recognized but has not been acknowledged, and it may occur at different times for each person respectively), they must find themselves alone together, and usually, they will have been drinking. These types of relationships will be addressed throughout this chapter. Finally, there is the romantic dating relationship, described here in more detail.

Romantic Relationships

In a romantic dating relationship, a couple may date for as much as a year before much sexual activity occurs, perhaps beginning in high school. In this case, heterosexual relationships develop slowly over time and trust is well established before sexual activity intensifies. Before first intercourse, the couple has typically been sexually active for a time, and the man has been urging the woman to go further. This situation is particularly true of first sexual relationships. There were seven participants with this type of pattern, where the first partners were people they had been dating since high school, and for four of them, with whom they were still involved. They were all heterosexual, four were Asian; one was Latina; one was African American; the other, a Caucasian man, came from a religious family. This was Eric, a freshman, and the only male participant who had not yet had genital intercourse. He felt some regret that sex had ultimately impinged on their friendship:

> I think the first time we had oral sex was the, yeah, it was this summer. It was like 7 months after we were going out, before the time when we became really close. And then we broke up and the first month or so

when we got back together, we didn't really do anything because it was the feeling-out period for both of us. And then we just started up and—I wouldn't say it was a routine thing, it didn't happen very often, you know, between us and stuff. We went probably, we started doing it maybe once a week or so—oral sex.

Eric explained how they handled the progression of their sexual feelings and activities.

Um, it was like—you know, the Bible says certain things about you know remaining a virgin until marriage and stuff like that. And so we would, when we would start getting closer, something like that then—we never did have sex—and we would start getting close or if something like that, it would always be like we would start getting like scared almost. But um, I think the biggest thing is communication.

DL: How did you talk about it?

Eric: Um, just like just open up, say what you feel, you know both sides. Let her talk, then I would say what I feel. Just say if we thought it was right, if we were ready for that. 'Cause I know, we'd been going out like 8 months, I think, and then that was the first time we got really really close to, you know, having sex and it was like—we stopped and just said "Let's talk about this," so we just sat down and talked. We just thought to each other and spoke to each other, and it just wasn't *right*, we weren't ready for it at the time, 'cause we were just going into our senior year in high school and we both weren't ready for it, we weren't ready to take that next step in the relationship. 'Cause we didn't feel that we were the greatest, you know, the bestest friends in the whole world.

They broke up shortly thereafter, and at the time of the interview, Eric was dating a more experienced woman who was taking the initiative. A follow-up interview may have told whether his resolve to remain a virgin lasted throughout his college career.

INTERCOURSE WITH FIRST PARTNERS

There were six participants who were still involved with their first partners, people with whom they had established trust over time. Four of these individuals were Asian, one was Latina, and one was African American. The couple may have talked about how they felt about sex beforehand, but none ever openly planned intercourse or contraception before the first time. In each case, the man had been asking to have sex for some time before the woman consented. They explained how the first times they had intercourse had happened. For Rita, being brought up by Asian parents made the decision difficult, one with which she wasn't entirely comfortable.

> DL: How did he know the first time? Did you decide in advance and talk about it? and say, "Okay, tonight's the night?"
>
> Rita: Kind of, yeah, because it was a big topic with us for a long time and we did talk about it for a long time. I don't know why I decided to do it. But it's kind of this thing I think back on it now and why I decided at that point I decided that it was okay. I don't think it was entirely okay for me.
>
> DL: Did you go pretty far before that?
>
> Rita: Umm, before I decided, yeah, we went pretty far. But I'm not really sure why I did it, besides the comfort level being . . . Like, after that year I knew him pretty well. Like he wasn't dating me just for sex. That was actually a main thing too for me.

Ginger was no longer seeing her first partner, but she remembered that before she had intercourse for the first time, she had been seeing a man for 4 months and had "been saying no for a long time." Her reaction was similar to Rita's. She felt ready but hadn't planned for sex that night, "I didn't have it like all planned out, but I thought any night when we got together could've been the night. But I just kept saying no, you know? And I, I really don't, wasn't sure *what* I would say at the moment. Right?" Like Rita, Ginger was ambivalent about her first time:

> I guess people tend to romanticize the idea of sex, and they have very high expectations as to what it's gonna be, it's like this dramatic thing that's gonna change your life. But especially when your parents tell you can only have sex with the one you marry. And it better be a strait-laced Asian engineer, right? So I, I thought um . . . you know, um no, it was good. But I, I was expecting something better, just because I'd been you know, just because the way people talk about sex, it's such a taboo, it's like something you, so, it's so . . . prohibited, you know? That you would expect it to be a big deal. But it wasn't a big deal. You know what I mean? I mean it felt good but it wasn't a big deal.

Charlie's girlfriend eventually became an enthusiastic and equal partner, but initially, intercourse was his idea.

DL: The first time, did you know it was gonna happen that day?

Charlie: No. I had no idea it was gonna happen that day. Um . . . Yeah, I had no idea it was gonna happen. Um, I didn't think it was gonna happen because she, she told me that she really didn't want to have sex before marriage, and I said okay, that's fine. I was willing to go with that. But then I think that day that it happened we were, we were you know going out for a long time without doing it, and I guess, I don't know, we just kept pushing ourselves to that point before we just did it, and not doing it—

DL: You mean that one time or for a series of times, going a little bit farther and farther?

Charlie: The first time. The very first time. We kept pushing ourselves without actually doing any penetration and she'd lie on top of me, but we didn't do anything until that minute, or I think . . . I think what happened was I asked her.

DL: If you could?

Charlie: Yeah. And at first, she was hesitant so we didn't for a couple minutes, and I asked her again. When I asked her again, she said, and I asked as if she . . . she said yes. I said, "Is it because you really want it?" And she said, "Yeah." So I penetrated her, and then after I pulled out, after the first penetration, I said, "Did it hurt?" and she said, "Yeah." So we stopped. Because it hurt her, so I, I didn't continue.

DL: Did you kind of feel like it was your place to ask and her place to decide?

Charlie: Well, I already knew *my* answer, because I knew I wanted to. But I didn't want to go, go ahead and just do it, I wanted her to, I wanted her to be able to say yes too. I didn't just want to do it. So um, I already knew my answer. I mean, 'cause she had asked me, 'cause if she had wanted it, I probably would have said yes. But I guess I asked her because um she always feels like I'm the one pushing, well at the beginning at least, she always felt like I was the one pushing. So she'd always stop me. And that was always fine with me.

DL: How did you feel to be viewed as the one pushing?

Charlie: Well, afterwards, it always seems bad, I always ask her, am I pushing her, 'cause she says sometimes that she thinks we're going too fast.

DL: Did you feel like you were pressuring her?

Charlie: Um . . . No, I didn't really think so, because you know, if she told me to stop I'd always back off, you know, and I didn't really think I was pressuring her, because she never like really was against anything I did, I mean she always enjoyed it, and I always ask her if, before I'd take like this big step, like before oral sex, I always asked her, if she wanted it, if she wanted to try it, or experiment, whatever. And she, she was pretty willing, and I guess now I'd say no because after the first couple times of sex she, also started taking a dominant role, she started requesting a lot of things. So, because she did that, um, you know, I don't feel . . .

DL: You felt like it was pretty equal.

Charlie: Yeah. Right now I don't feel like I pressured her because right now she asks for a lot of things, too.

Sonia, a Latina, was emotionally ready for her first time, although her partner didn't know that it would be that night.

Sonia: I don't know, I just felt like I did. I mean I . . . I don't know. I mean I felt ready. I don't know *why* I felt ready, but it just, I felt comfortable with him, I guess.

DL: With this one.

Sonia: Mm-hm.

DL: He was the first one?

Sonia: Yeah, with my husband. I just felt really comfortable with him, and there was more communication between me and him. Like we talked just about everything. I mean we talked about sex before we even had sex.

DL: What did you talk about? About it.

Sonia: Just about, you know, how I would feel because he was a virgin also. He hadn't had sex with anybody else. So we would just talk about oh, what it would be like, or when we planned to lose our virginity, or with who, and things like that. And I mean I've never talked to other guys you know about sex in that way. And . . . or I just felt really comfortable with him.

DL: So after you had been dating for a while, that's when you started talking about it?

Sonia: No, actually before. When we were just talking on the phone, yeah. We were just getting to know each other. Then—I mean 'cause when we started talking, it seemed like we already knew each other kind of, 'cause we had a lot of things in common. And then . . . And we were just, we would just talk about everything. We'd stay up 'til 3 or 4 in the morning just talking about all kinds of things. And then this was like at the beginning of our senior year, and we didn't start going out 'til like December. 'Cause we started talking in about August or July of '89. That's when we started getting really close. And we started going out, going to the movies or things like that or whatever, 'til December. And then we didn't start getting intimate, having any sexual intercourse until April of '90.

DL: How did that proceed? A little bit at a time, or . . . ?

Sonia: Yeah. We did um . . . We didn't start kissing until like February. And then—

DL: So [it was] 3 months before you kissed each other?

Sonia: Mm-hm. And then afterwards then we started, then he came coming around the house a lot of times, and we would kiss and everything, and . . . And then there were times when he would come by and my parents weren't there. Because my senior year, they started having teacher in-service days, where we had Mondays off or something. Like one Monday a month or something off. And so he would come by the house those days, and nobody else was there because my mother was away in college and my little brother and sister, they still had school. So I was there by myself and he would come and see me. And we would kiss and everything. And then eventually it just evolved you know, until we had you know, we had sexual intercourse in my parents' house on one of those days, too, I think it was. Yeah. On one of those teacher in-service days, in April.

DL: So before, did you, how did you decide that time that that was going to be the time?

Sonia: We didn't. We didn't plan that you know that day was gonna be It, but we tried to have sexual intercourse before. But you know, since we were both inexperienced, we couldn't do anything. I mean it took a while. It took practice until finally we succeeded.

Within these couples, a pattern was established where a woman decided generally that she was ready to move their sexual practice to the next stage, but it wasn't planned so carefully that she decided on the first time in advance.

PUTTING ON THE BRAKES

Among all those I interviewed who were still involved with their first partners, the woman decided when intercourse would occur the first time, didn't tell the man in advance, yet the man was assumed to be willing and expected to be equipped with the condom.

Sarita: Yeah I could, yeah but I didn't want to go through that. So um my whole thing was oh gosh, I can't get pregnant. So, and then what I even thought was, or what I had been taught was um if you use a condom, you won't get pregnant. And I didn't know much about condoms, but the first time, let's see, the first time I had intercourse was with the guy that I was going out with in high school. And he had come up to visit, and I'd always held back, and I guess I was just ready. And we used a condom.

DL: Who had it?

Sarita: Um, he did.

DL: Did you talk about it before he came up?

Sarita: Um, I guess just right before I said.

DL: Before he came up for the weekend did you say?

Sarita: Yeah. Oh before? Nonono. No. Um, I hadn't, I hadn't, I hadn't planned it. I mean I hadn't said, okay, you come up for the weekend, now—we're going to have sex?

DL: Did you say it to yourself?

Sarita: Um . . . I think it crossed my mind, yeah. I thought oh it could probably you know it could finally happen this weekend. And I didn't—But I didn't think about contraception at the time, I mean I didn't prepare for it, I didn't go out and get a condom or I didn't do anything like that. And then when he came to visit um we started getting physical like we usually did, and then I guess I just didn't stop it this time.

DL: So that was your job to decide when to move further?

Sarita: Yeah. Yeah, it was my job to—I mean he, I mean I knew for a while that he had wanted to go further but I would always just stop and say look, this is, I'm just not comfortable, or um, I can't. And he was really understanding, he wouldn't force it or anything. Um, he, he, he'd just always say, "Okay, well, as long as you tell me," and that kind of thing. . . . So I just didn't stop him, but I was really embarrassed to talk about even though I had known him for a while, I was really embarrassed to talk about, like I knew I wanted him to put on the condom but I didn't know how to say it? Um, and I was kind of hoping that he would just pick it up out of somewhere. . . .

Mary's first and only sexual relationship was characterized by ambivalence and also a certain passivity. She and Theresa were the least interested in sex among those I interviewed. Unlike the others, Mary expressed neither desire or enthusiasm, even in retrospect.

Yeah. We were just like, you know, doing the whole kissing, whole petting thing. And then . . . 'Cause he was, he was very persistent. So that was the one thing, 'cause he'd tried before, and he was just very, very persistent. And I would always stop him but then this one time I just didn't stop him.

The romantic relationship is prototypical of women's responsibility to control the progression of sexual activity. Men attempt to bring the sexual activity to the next level, and women must—often literally—hold them back.

DISCONTINUING CONDOMS AFTER TRUST IS ESTABLISHED

In the romantic relationship, a woman is usually willing to use oral contraceptives when trust has been established. Denise, Lauren, Hanan, Susannah, and Sarita used or would consider the pill:

Sarita: Right. So it's only been a year since, or a little over a year ago that this was, that I actually decided that I was thinking about the pill. And that was only because I knew that we were in a monogamous relationship and I would never I mean if I was on the pill and I was having sex with someone I didn't know very well or anyone else, I mean I just would use a condom anyway. Because now I know about STDs. But um, so we decided that I mean actually I brought up that maybe, you know, why don't I go on the pill, it would be a lot nicer I think.

Even though she might consider being on the pill, Hanan didn't have sufficient trust to eschew condoms in her current relationship:

That would just be a trust issue, and for me, for the most part, even if I did go on the pill, I would still be using condoms. I think if I go on the pill, it's my decision, and my body, and I don't even know, I mean in this relationship, I would tell him, yeah, I'm gonna be on the pill, but we're still gonna use condoms.

Sebastian imagined a romantic relationship where he would eventually be able to go without condoms but had learned about the danger of trust from his previous relationship. He added a note of caution after he'd found his partner had been with another man. He was forced to consider the parameters of such a relationship in more concrete terms. He thought he would like to start off using a condom, [be] involved with them long enough that they would need to um . . . In my terms of long enough are like 5 years at least. I mean I'm talking long time now. And . . . 'Cause I know the situations, and I think it at least takes me 5 years to get to know someone well enough to trust 'em. A year or 2 isn't long enough. I mean I think when you're on 3 or 4 years, you've pretty much, you know, can guess but, I mean, I'm talking about those things.

Denise felt she had reached that point with her partner, "'cause we're at the point where we're so honest with each other,"

Well I mean, see, we always care about each other, but sometimes, like if one of us, if one of us had met a guy and you know we started going out and stuff, and we want to um pursue a sexual relationship with this person, unless we give each other the freedom to do it, just because we're both at a part where we really don't know. I mean it's hard being bisexual, because, it's just, you don't know. Because it's like we care about each other, but we also, if we find a man, we care about them too, and it's really hard to negotiate all that, and to negotiate your feelings. So it's kind of like right now we're trying to be really open with each other so we don't stifle ourselves into being one way because right now we're still growing. . . . We go out to straight bars and flirt with guys or we'll decide one night that we want to go to, like, a Castro bar and just hang out and be ourselves and talk just to ourselves. . . . The weird thing is is that we have never at any time gone with, or tried another partner that was a woman. It's always been men. Because it's kind of like we know as two women we're almost perfect.

Denise was unique in this respect; for her, it was honesty more than monogamy that was essential to trust in her relationship. Although she felt committed to her partner, she was aware that her sexuality was still in process and that the relationship might have room for outside experimentation for either of them.

COMMITMENT AND TRUST

After establishing an exclusive relationship, a couple evaluates it by discussing whether they want to be "in a commitment." Charlie described the difference between a more casual relationship and a committed one:

All my friends who've slept with a girl say after you sleep with a girl, you know, there's nothing really left, you know, you can't explore anything more. There's nothing more to look forward to. And that's when you really tell if you care for the girl when—beyond physical feelings. If you can have sex with a girl and still feel for her afterwards, then you got a thing better than if you just slept with her. Which is why I say a lot of people after they sleep once together they start pulling away. And that's, that's how they judge.

For Lauren, knowing the status of her relationship was important to help decide whether to pursue a relationship with another man who interested her:

Lauren: We've been on basically for the past 10 months, but we haven't been in a commitment, but ever since the first month, it's been pretty much exclusive, just the two of us.

DL: So the commitment is something that people usually do officially?

Lauren: Well, it is a commitment, but just the word's not there. 'Cause I told him, I said, "Okay, if we're not in a commitment, [and] you get together with anybody else, it's over." So it is a commitment, but it's just the word's not there like I want you to be my girlfriend, I want you to be my boyfriend.

DL: So is that the big issue between you is you want a commitment and he doesn't want one?

Lauren: Yeah. Yeah, but it's not that he doesn't want one, it's just he's a really private person, he's just not sure if he's ready for it or not, so last night I just said I'm not waiting any more, that's it.

DL: But he hasn't been seeing anybody else?

Lauren: No. It's kind of that, 'cause it's just, it's almost like it's a good relationship, I just want the security of knowing that it's exclusive between us.

For Leo, his present relationship came too quickly after the last one to get serious, "yeah, we haven't established anything major in terms of a commitment to each other. The word did come up, something along those lines. And it's so absurd, [after] 3 weeks." Raphael's partner tried to ascertain the kind of relationship he wanted,

He just asked me, "have you been dating anybody else or are you just wanting a fling, or . . . ?" And I told him I was looking for a relationship and he asked me why, and I said because I'm tired of the other.

Wheeler and his current partner had the discussion after 3 or 4 weeks: "I was and he was being monogamous too, even though we had never really talked about monogamy, or even though we didn't consider ourselves to be in a relationship, the discussion kind of progressed from there." Between men, the only difference I noticed was a greater fluidity in reference to the length of time they needed to call something a relationship: Leo and Wheeler thought about commitment after seeing a man for 3 weeks; Raphael referred to risk in the context of "if it's gonna be a really short relationship like 1 day or something . . . "

For Shawn, his partner's pushing the envelope led to him ending the relationship:

> I really liked this girl a lot, but I wanted to like, you know, just be really relaxed right now with our relationship, not get too intense, and that kind of stuff, and it's not like I've been seeing a lot of other people right now just because I've been so busy, and so I said, you know, well let's just take it easy and she's like oh well either we break up or we could continue to go out but I can't have any gray areas here, so I said okay, well, I guess we'll just have to break up, you know, 'cause that's not what I really want, but you know I don't want to put myself in a bad situation here, or so anyway, I wanted to break up a little bit before I left for the summer so we'd both feel, it wouldn't be like we'd be going out and then just split, and I thought that would be harder if we just did that than if we kinda tapered down. And that's what she didn't understand.

One's perception of risk is related to real or perceived risk factors but also to the level of trust in the relationship. All relationships, in contrast to casual liaisons, are founded on trust. As long as the expectation of monogamy is part of that trust, one cannot reconcile protecting oneself as though the partner were mistrusted. For young women particularly, the construction of trust exists in symbiotic relation to the notions of both *commitment* and *relationship*. Trust usually implies exclusivity and always, safety. As other authors have noted (Hein, 1988; Holland, Ramazanoglu, Scott, Sharpe, et al., 1990; Moore & Rosenthal, 1993), young people's typical patterns of serial monogamy by no means offer protection from either STDs or heartbreak.

Gender and Sexual Orientation Differences in Relationships

Both men and women interested in having a romantic relationship want one based on friendship; however, their ideas about what constitutes friendship differ somewhat. Men wanted a sexual companion, "why most guys want relationships, well, after the physical part at the beginning, is because they just want someone to do something with" (Charlie). "We were able to have oral sex or foreplay or do whatever, you know, just screw around and then be able to go outside and have a water fight. Or, just, you know, just fun stuff like you do with your best friend" (Eric). Andrew's girlfriend

> is a great friend to have. And one of the things that attracted me the most is I have a really strange sense of humor . . . she not only laughs at it, she participates in it. . . . And she is very smart and very liberal and open-minded.

Women's definition of friendship seemed to be based more on communication. Susannah succinctly expressed what most of the women said:

> Now I want something stable, I want someone to be there. I want to be able to talk to you about things and if you can't do that, then I'm going to find somebody else who can do those things. Because that's what I want. I want a good friendship with the added sexual relationship and I want it all to be good.

For Denise, the gender difference in values would probably lead to her becoming lesbian eventually:

> Yeah, the monogamy issue's always a problem and we always, I mean . . . see for me it, it's developed into, if I find, if I even, it gets harder and harder as we are together more and more to even find a man that I would want to have sex with because I would demand so much more than just having it be sex. Because I want someone that's gonna be, you know, emotionally in sync with me.

Where women wanted a soul mate, men wanted a pal. Some of the men, notably Charlie and Andrew, told of relationships that were just as important to them as they were to women. Yet because men operate differently than women in relationships, men are seen as being less invested. The qualities that were valued were different for women but not necessarily better or worse than men's. Because women have traditionally been viewed as the keepers of the relationship, women get to define what constitutes its necessary elements.

THE CHALLENGE OF ACKNOWLEDGING DESIRE

Both men and women are aware that women risk their reputations if they acknowledge their sexual desires; on the other hand, there is little awareness on the part of either sex of the impact of sexual relations on men's emotional lives. Women can't tell their partners they want sex because of what they have been taught about the physical and emotional risks involved and the messages they have received about appropriate behavior for young women. When they get to university, often they quite consciously attempt to leave their conditioning behind:

> Ginger: You know, when I first came to Berkeley, it was just all social. I didn't do anything. I didn't, I didn't—there's no studying, there's no books—What are you *talking* about, it's my freshman year! And so I was just seeing a lot of people, I was meeting a lot of people, and um . . . And I just would only go a certain point, and then it goes farther and farther. And I kept thinking, why am I saying no, right? Because I've been conditioned to say no, you know, because my *parents* are telling me to say no. Then well what—I need to think for myself, right? I mean, what's going on here? And there was no reason. I had, I could give myself no reason to say no. So that was it.

However, even though they come to permit desire, they have no language with which to discuss it. Ann gave me an example of "scripted refusal" (Muehlenhard & McCoy, 1991) in a sexual experience where she had explained to a partner,

> You can stay but, you know, we've got our ground rules here. You stay on your side and I'll stay on my side." But then, within a matter of minutes, that was just like . . . it wasn't a very sincere ground rule to begin with.

She had felt obliged to pretend she didn't want or intend to have sex because she felt it was expected in the situation.

THE "MISSING DISCOURSE OF DESIRE"

Until the consolidation of sexual progress of which Keller et al. (1982) wrote occurs, one finds a continued construction of young women as sexual targets fighting off the uncontrolled and uncontrollable lust of young men. Adolescent girls have little opportunity to explore or act on their own desire and sexuality in this view (Fine, 1988). Michelle Fine notes that,

> educated primarily as the potential victims of male sexuality, women represent no subject in their own right. Young women are still taught to fear and defend in isolation from exploring desire, and in this context there is little possibility of their developing a critique of gender or sexual arrangements. (p. 30)

She has called the censure of a positive view of women's sexuality "the missing discourse of desire." She argues that the constriction of a male-defined sexuality allows women only one response, "yes or no—to a question that is not necessarily their own. A discourse of desire in which young women have a voice would be informed and generated out of their own socially constructed sexual meanings" (p. 34).

As discussed earlier, high school curricula portray sexuality as alternately violent, victimizing, and a reflection of individual morality. Fine (1988) contends that a discourse of female desire, pleasure, or sexual entitlement is missing for high school girls; however,

> a discourse of desire, although absent in the 'official' curriculum, is by no means missing from the lived experiences or commentaries of young women. Their struggle to untangle issues of gender, power, and sexuality underscores the fact that notions of sexual negotiation are not separated from sacrifice and nurture for them. (p. 35)

This situation is only partly ameliorated by the time young people start university.

DESIRE AND REPUTATION

The repercussions for women who act on their desire are reflected in the language. I was disappointed to learn that the double standard is alive and well. Women who have too many partners are called "sluts" or "'hos" (whores), but men are "players" or "studs." The words for sexually experienced women are universally considered derogatory, whereas those for men are not.

> Sarita: Another thing we talked about in our section was that females are kind of taught to, if females have a lot of sexual encounters they're looked upon as sluts whereas if males do, they're looked upon as kind of studs or—
>
> DL: Even these days men are . . . ?

Sarita: Even these days, yeah, definitely. And that was one of the big things we talked about in section. So I think females have to have some sort of scapegoat as to why. Or they have to justify why they're being sexually active. Not only to other people but to their friends, I mean not only to their friends but to themselves is what I meant. Um . . . Just because yeah, I think that there's all this little bit of guilt because of what society says.

Other participants elaborated—apparently, it is more damaging in the eyes of friends and community that a lot of people know that a woman has many partners.

DL: How many is "sleeping around"? How many does it take to be sleeping around?

Joseph: I don't know. Knowledge, I guess. I'm sure people've slept around, but if, if you and your friends know about it,

DL: So that's something that's defined externally.

Joseph: That's known, yeah. Something that's known.

Vicky: Okay. Well, let me talk about her first, I guess, it's hard for me to generalize. Well, for her, she went out with . . . there's a group of really close guys. She slept with all of them, so to me, that's a 'ho. I mean to sleep with . . . I mean it's like . . .

As George illustrates later, even in the age of AIDS, men are not normally vilified for their number of sexual partners by either other men or women. Quite the opposite, according to some:

DL: So if a woman thought a man had too many partners, what would he be called? What's the equivalent to a whore or a slut?

George: Probably a stud, he's good in bed, he's popular.

Rita: I found out later from other people that he's a big player.

DL: Does that mean he has a lot of partners?

Rita: Yeah. A lot of girls think that he has a really awesome body sort of thing and everything. So a lot of girls do consent to it.

Joseph thought a "player is someone who charms girls, and just has a certain arrogance to him." I asked him about the word *stud*, which he defined as "a good-looking guy I guess. That a lot of girls like." However, some of Joseph's female friends are evocatively attempting to reclaim the language, and Joseph accords them the same status as male friends:

> See, they call themselves "The *PUTAs.*"[1] It's an abbreviation. *Proud United Tramp Association.* I don't know why they call themselves that. They're not, they're not. Some of them have messed around with some guys, um, I don't think no more than guys have.

George illustrated how attitudes about sexually active women have been codified:

> There are girls for example, there's girls in sororities that we put on what is called "The List." If more than three guys or three guys or more guys had sex with a certain girl, then they're put on a list and only we know where the list is. Okay, and that's a way of kind of socializing around sex, but you have to look at *why* this girl would go out and have sex with three different guys in the same fraternity. You just can't look at the attitude that the men have, you have to look at where and why their attitude *is* like that, if it would come from a certain girl, now the girl might not be a whore, she might not be a slut, or she might not *be* this person, but she's had sex with three or more guys, and in our eyes that's what, you know, she's on The List. She's classified as that.

In addition to this public censure, George did his part to preserve the traditional order within his own relationships. George was no anomaly, for although his attitude was the most extreme of all the participants, it was by no means unusual. I was distressed that George held a position of influence as a section leader in the health education class from which I had recruited participants, although he was oblivious to both the irony of his remarks and any reaction I might have to them. Consider the difference in attitude regarding a male friend and a female potential partner:

> George: I have a friend, who I consider a good friend, his name is Brad, he's probably had sex with probably about over a hundred women and he had sex when he was 15.
>
> DL: He's around your age?
>
> George: Yeah. He's 22. And it's really funny because he doesn't practice safe sex all the time. He's gotten a couple STDs, he knows about the AIDS thing, he knows that this is what he should be doing, but he doesn't, it's something that just comes.

Though he knew his views weren't consistent across gender, he continued:

> George: I've kind of made a decision in my life that whatever relationship I get into it's going to be ideal and you know I'm going to work with somebody. Like I met this girl, not this girl, but I met this other girl a couple of months ago and she couldn't communicate, she couldn't talk. She . . . basically we started talking, see that's a whole 'nother thing, you could like somebody, you could be attracted to them and have you start finding out about their past sexual history and you're just like, whoa, wait a minute, this girl is basically told me she had four abortions and I was just, well, you know. I don't want to classify you into a certain category but I know from my perspective that I don't want to get into that type of relationship, you've had that type of experience and I don't think that that's—I told her that, I kind of said that I don't want you to, I don't want to get into with her as a relationship.
>
> DL: What does that imply to you, about having four abortions?
>
> George: Where her morals are. Where her ideas about safe sex come from. What she's thinking about, what goes on through her head, why, and her explanation to me was she went to the doctor. And the doctor explained to her that she was very fertile and I said, "Okay, well that's fine, now you tell me the times you got pregnant." And she said, "Well, the first time, we used a condom and still got pregnant," and I said, "Okay, well what happened?" She said, "I don't know, we didn't really talk about it, I just got pregnant and I had an abortion, the second time I was using a fertility awareness method," and I said, "You know, unless you incorporate and you're really really accurate, it's not probably the safest way to go about things," and she said, "Well, I wasn't really accurate and I used it anyway and I got pregnant," and then she said, "The third time I was just stupid, and I wasn't thinking and I didn't use any type of protection at all and I got pregnant." After she got done explaining this to me, I was just like, what are you thinking? I said, "I feel sorry for you if you cannot have the morals and the values to think about what you've done and what's gone on in your life." I mean *four* abortions. There's something going on there. How do you feel, how does it make you feel where's your self esteem, where's your balance, where's your empowerment, are you questioning what you're doing, and she couldn't and all of a sudden, I realized . . .
>
> DL: So when you think of *that* woman and how you felt about her—I realize that she was a prospective partner, but then you also talked

about your friend—is there a difference about how you think about their morals or values?

George: Yeah, one's a male and one's a female.

DL: What about it?

George: And where those roles come in. Umm . . . 'cause one of the guys, the guy is my friend, he's someone I grew up with and I've kind of understood and related that this is my friend and when we go out we have fun together and we do things and maybe some of the stereotypes of what men are in society and what women are and if the man goes out and gets all these women and that's fine—'cause him and I can sit and we can talk about the experiences and he can sit there and tell me what happened and who he was with and all that great stuff and I could go, okay that's fine, that's great. I don't preach to him, I don't say, well, maybe you should do this, or what's going on. But with *her*, I almost find it necessary to say, you know, I feel like, I don't know, I feel like she should know what's going on, because she's a woman and she's the one that had four abortions and I think in my mind having four abortions versus going out and having protected sex or unprotected sex like this guy is, I think the four abortions maybe is little harsher, you know, I feel like, I just don't want, and another thing is too, her and I could still be friends but I don't want any kind of romantic between that, but this guy and myself are friends and we're heterosexual friends and there's no way, I don't have to worry . . .

Denise's experience as a sorority member was an exception to the reputation management of women. According to her, the sororities have their own list, one where it is considered positive to have multiple sexual partners. As a member, Denise disapproved of the sexual competition, even disliked the pressure so much that she left; however, she didn't disparage the women for their sexuality:

We both ended up moving out of the sorority because people started talking 'cause we weren't doing everything sorority girls are supposed to do, we hung out with each other mostly. So I dropped out.

DL: What weren't you doing?

Denise: I wasn't going out and screwing every other guy and . . .

DL: Is that what sorority girls were doing?

Denise: Oh yeah. When I was a pledge, that was the biggest problem. We had a chart on the door and all the houses, they'd line up all the fraternities and then they had a chart where your name was on it for how many guys you slept with in that sorority, they'd put a mark there and my mark there was nothing there.

In spite of the sexual competition at her sorority, even Denise found rules of gender behavior to be socially constructed. The rules also vary by type of relationship. Midwinter (1992) found that the greatest sex differences occur in situations involving a romantic interest, where rules require that males be more direct than females in pursuing that interest. Rules for directness of approach prescribe different behavior for men and women, which accord with previous findings of male instrumentality and female expressiveness and that the gender-specific rules for directness of approach have most relevance to romantic situations. Though George, quoted earlier, is a flagrant example, Wight (1992), too, still found stigma associated with women carrying condoms and a conflation of unrepressed female sexuality with worthlessness and dirt. The Women Risk and AIDS Project (Holland, Ramazanoglu, Scott, et al., 1991; Holland, Ramazanoglu, Sharpe, et al., 1991) discussed earlier and the work of the researchers at the Australian National Centre in HIV Social Research (Kippax, Crawford, & Waldby, 1994; Kippax, Crawford, Waldby, & Benton, 1990) reinforces the findings here, that women are still seen as the objects of desire and risk censure when they attempt to explore their own sexual subjectivity.

GENDER AND POWER

When women experiment with their sexual power at university, reactions vary from support to censure. One of the women on Hanan's dorm floor

was just very . . . she was aware of her body and I guess what she could do, use, do with it. You know, that she had a nice body. I mean she was skinny, to me she was just really skinny, but some people are attracted to that you know, she was just very flirtatious and if someone gave her a sign that they were interested, she would just go with it. She was just very oversexed.

Although Hanan disapproved of a woman using her sexuality in this way, she was extremely aware of her own power. Hanan came across as both powerful and traditional. Her feminine values were reflected in her belief about appropriate gender roles.

I did crush a few men who were weaker, personality wise. Because I would dominate, and I would, I guess I have a slight power trip too, also. So sometimes I'll test people to see what they'll do. . . . It was like, "I don't want to run this relationship. It's supposed to be equal."

Shawn and Vicky were each other's gender counterparts among the participants, viewing relationship issues from a similar stereotypical position. As did the men in the Men Risk and AIDS study (Holland, Ramazanoglu, Sharpe, & Thomson, 1994), Shawn reacted to power struggle by making himself less vulnerable:

> When I broke up, broke up with my ex-girlfriend, it made me all the more stronger in terms of going out with other people. I was able to just, never really become attached to them and go out and have a great time with them, and give a lot, but not become attached to them. And I would just, I would always have the upper hand in that relationship, in most relationships.

Both he and Vicky approached conflict and power in relationships like training a dog, using the expression *whipped* to describe someone caring about them. Shawn was ambivalent about ending the relationship, both regretful and angry. As illustrated earlier in the discussion about women's reputations, one's sexual relationships are constructed with friends as well as lovers. Part of what is important about the balance of power in a relationship concerns how friends perceive it.

> Shawn: So when I broke up with her Friday, the next day we had a party at my fraternity house and she came over to the party, she hung out all day at the party and stuff. Drove me crazy. She didn't talk to me all day long, talked to other guys and stuff right in front of me and then just hung out with this one guy all day long. Even though I knew that she was whipped on me she just, she just kind of sat there to like just to, to show me you know well okay if you're going to let me go then I'm going to go on with my life. And I just said, "Oh God. What the hell did I do?" That really ticked me off.

> Vicky: I don't think public affection is bad, just like not like too extreme but I think it's good. It shows, especially when a guy does it, it shows other people, "I'm not whupped, I just care for her," because guys don't show public affection 'cause their guy friends think, "yeah, you're whupped on her" and you know, "she has you by the leash" and it's this whole thing what your friends think . . .

So although Vicky understood that public perception was important, she used her power in an ultrafeminine way to keep her partner in his place. I had an image of her with a rolled up newspaper as she described their first intercourse:

> He was like trained already, you know [laughs], and he stopped and I didn't stop him but I could tell he hesitated and he hesitated because he was shocked I didn't stop and I think it was a shock to him, so see that's—I think that's the purpose of that whole power thing where see, if you don't have—not necessarily power over him—but not control, but just sort of, you have to discipline them sometimes where you have to show them that I mean that it makes it something special where it's like, oh, you know, "This is it, she didn't stop me," and it makes it more exciting than just like reaching over the first time, getting the condom and then like, "I am a man" sort of thing so I think it helps a lot, um, especially with a guy like that who has—not necessarily a big ego but who—I guess he does kind of have a big ego. I don't know how to explain it. You have to—with some guys where they are more understanding and more I think it has a lot to do with being a male chauvinist because a lot of the girls I know that are very dominant in the relationship, they are able to talk to their boyfriend about anything, everything, whereas where somebody is more dominant, that has more of an ego, that's where you have to play even harder to get—with their ego—if that makes any sense.

In the discourse on gender, both men and women are aware of a man's "need to prove his manhood" (Holland et al., 1994, p. 143). In Vicky's case, she used her position as a virgin to take control of that discourse, whereas Shawn contributes to the construction of what Holland and colleagues call the assumption of a "hegemonic masculinity" to manage his vulnerability.

SEXUALITY AND GENDER IN PROCESS

Sexuality is processual rather than static at this age, and many participants found themselves changing while at university. In spite of her feminist orientation, Janice felt disempowered by and ashamed of her response to her partner's resistance to contraception, "And here I am, a big strong woman, I don't have to deal with that. I tell men where to go . . . then here I am now involved in this deep relationship and it's still . . . I still feel like that." As a result, she found herself becoming attracted to Andre, whom she perceived to be more egalitarian. Lauren found herself feeling more assertive in response to the feminist ideas to which she'd been exposed at Berkeley:

I took a women's studies class last semester, too. Last semester was just my sex class, my women's studies, my *bam*. Um. I think it has 'cause it's gotten me to know that I have just as much power as the guy. I have the right to say no, and if I want to have sex, I should be able to have sex. It isn't like guys are supposed to have sex, girls're supposed to wait. It's like if I wanta have sex, I'm gonna have sex. And so, it's given me more of like this, well I'm gonna do it if I wanta do it, but if I don't wanta do it, I'm not gonna do it. And I'm not gonna say, "Oh well, you just gotta please the guys."

Denise didn't understand men's continuing sexism, "unless it's just this whole idea that they really hate women." She felt more confident as a result of her relationship with Maritza:

I don't know if it's because I've had relationships with women, but it's really easy for me to be, I mean this is something new, too, because it's been like a growing process for me the last 3 years but growing and you know thinking about sexual roles, it's easy for me to approach a man and deal with the whole issues. I feel stronger, actually.

She felt that "women are getting a little bit, although I don't know what statistics say, myself and people I know, seem to be getting more stronger about being assertive, I think."

Susannah wanted to think she was better prepared to ask for what she wanted:

If I were to go out now, and pursue something sexual with somebody, I would probably be more inclined maybe to ask more questions than I had done in the past. About what sexual things that they had done, who they had been with, and probably not too soon that they've already been with opposite sex people. Whereas, I don't think I would have thought about that as much as 5 years ago.

Even though mores were for the most part still very traditional, a few women had made progress toward expressing desire, and a few men had come to expect their partners to be equal in their sexual demands.

Note

1. A clever pun, because *puta* is Spanish slang for *whore*.

5

Risk and Trust in Relationships

We turn now to how risk and trust are constructed in sexual relationships. Participants varied widely in the amount of thought and practice they had put into negotiating sexual relationships in general and safer sex in particular. Risk was constructed on the basis of knowledge about transmission of sexually transmissible diseases (including HIV), the perceived safety of a partner or potential partner, and the context in which people met. The dominant epidemiological model of risk was generally not questioned. Trust was determined, especially for women, by the extent to which the relationship was considered exclusive. For the reasons discussed earlier and to be explored further, couples found it difficult to discuss each other's respective sexual histories and to acknowledge that they planned to have sex. Furthermore, some denied that their behaviors were risky or that they had power to change their situations.

The Construction of Trust

The perception of risk and trust were inversely related, opposite sides of the same coin. Partners who didn't know each other well in the beginning had legitimate grounds to behave as though a partner posed risk, though this usually occurred without acknowledgment between them, because the romantic discourse on sex presents it as an act between people in love. The transition from dating to relationship becomes a declaration of trust that implies honesty, fidelity, and nearly always, monogamy. Once monogamy is assumed, condoms as a symbol of risk and protection against one's lover must be overtly renegotiated as a means of contraception or discarded in favor of more effective methods. In either case, it is impossible to trust a partner, a lover, and simultaneously behave as though one or the other poses risk. Thus, both risk and trust were constructed in the process of selecting and getting to know a partner. On the basis of this information, people weighed the benefits of practicing safer sex with its inconvenience, when they thought about it at all. Thus, a gay man might decide that fellatio without ejaculation was safe enough when considering the taste of condoms; a woman might decide she could allow her male partner to forego condoms because she believed him monogamous. As long as nothing interfered with that construction, a person continued feeling safe with his or her choices. Evidence of a partner's nonmonogamy, a sexually transmitted disease, or even gaining new health information could alter the checks and balances of risk assessment.

EVALUATION OF POTENTIAL PARTNERS

Potential partners were sometimes assessed in terms of risk by their appearance or lifestyle characteristics. Men, both gay and straight, used this method more often than women to evaluate partners, even when they knew the approach to be irrational. They considered a potential partner's appearance, family background, place of origin, concern and knowledge about HIV, even daily schedule, to decide whether a partner presented a risk. "I sort of evaluate it and I sort of judge the people—I know this is wrong, it's like well, he *looks* like he might be disease free" (Dave). The concept of cleanliness was linked to lack of disease: "How clean, just even smells or body" (Donald), or "there's some girls that are just really beautiful and just really clean-cut and everything that you can tell" (Eric). They might try to verify their impression through friends, "finding out a little bit about them from other people" (Joseph), though at times finding their assumption incorrect: "I asked him afterwards and he said that she had been with a bunch of guys" (Eric). Donald believed a new partner, who said he'd tested negative, because of his demeanor:

> DL: So how do you decide whether to believe it or not, considering he picked you up on the street?

Donald: Um . . . It's just what I know about the person. He's . . . He's very, in this particular case he was very motivated and very um in his profession and into his life, and I just . . . I mean he was very cautious, also. He was very . . . He paid attention to detail and stuff like that, so I just—for me that said that he actually wanted to know or did figure I'd find out and was being careful about it, and that particular instance I was pretty confident that he was, you know, being truthful, just because of what I know about the person. He was very um . . . Like I said he was very motivated and into his life so . . .

DL: Could you see somebody lying or have you ever . . . ?

Donald: Could I see someone lying? He actually told me another reason I think I may have believed him is because he told me he had wan— he was very um he, he was always making sure that I knew what I was getting involved with and telling me that, you know, "You need to be careful, a lot of people will lie to you, blah-blah-blah, you have to make sure you know what you're getting into." Stuff like that. And I trusted him, so I mean I saw that he, you know, he was—he wasn't talking about himself when he said "You have to watch out who you're talking to and that some people lie, and I think he had a genuine interest in me as a person.

Sebastian had trusted his partner similarly:

DL: And you felt like he wasn't sexual with anybody else?

Sebastian: No.

DL: And um . . . What were the circumstances that led you to believe that? Because people lie, so how did you decide that you could trust that?

Sebastian: Oh yeah. Um . . . I just thought I could trust him, what he told me in talking to him, knowing his house situation and how he, like, knowing his schedule and stuff like that, it doesn't mean anything, they're just the little things that I use to determine . . .

DL: Oh, I'm asking you what they are.

Sebastian: Yeah. Um . . . He would travel a lot, and work a lot, work long hours and stuff. And being at the company I knew that was true, I mean I knew what he does and how much work he does do. But um, and so that's what I went on, and just pure trust.

DL: So what made you think he wasn't, you know, going to bars when he was travelling?

Sebastian: Oh, I'm sure, he might have been.

DL: Picking somebody up, I mean.

Sebastian: Yeah, yeah. He might have been. Um . . . 'Cause I saw what he was telling me and I just, that's, just . . .

DL: Did you have any agreement that, did you ever say, "If you're ever with somebody else I want you to tell me," or "if you're ever with somebody else I want you to not do these behaviors . . . "

Sebastian: I said that when we first got together, I said if any of us has any relationship with anyone else, I feel it's a right to tell the other person. I feel it has to be that way. In the very beginning, we spent the day together and we were sitting on the beach and I told him this.

DL: And he agreed to that?

Sebastian: Yeah. And we went over the whole AIDS issue again, and talked about it again, and he said what he'd said before, and he agreed to that, and um, so that was established then. That was that.

Sebastian later learned that his partner had not been monogamous, in an incident that influenced the way he would construct trust in the future.

Sebastian: See, there was an incidence . . . After we broke up I had come down to L.A. A couple times I had different things to do in L.A, and um one of the times we got together one day. And we were going up and down and our relationship was up and down. He really wasn't sure, and I of course was still very much in love with him, and um independent but also like desperately wanting to get back together in the sense of I would like to see you. I mean, I had, you know, but if that's if, what you decide, and stuff, but I had to like talk about it first of all, whatever. Anyway, so sometimes we were together, sometimes we were really separated. And then um I'd come down. We'd spent the night together. Um, the next morning I looked, I was getting ready to leave, and on his floor was a condom wrapper kind of coming out from the bed. And we hadn't used one the night before. And that, I just blew up. I mean it's great yes he's using condoms, that's fantastic, but . . . .

DL: But he was supposed to have told you.

Sebastian: The point is I didn't know. He didn't tell me. And so that was interesting.

DL: How'd you feel?

Sebastian: Betrayed. Very scared.

DL: Scared for . . . ?

Sebastian: Scared for my safety, betrayed for him lying. All of a sudden just like, "you're such an idiot, you know, for trusting someone to that extent." Um, and it all just hit me right there. And so we got in the car and I said, "Who've you been with?" I didn't ask *if* or anything. I said, "Who've have you been with?" And he knew. He knew that I knew. 'Cause I just, I went and looked right at him, and said, "Who have you been with?" And he stopped. I said, "Who have you slept with?" And he says, "I haven't *slept* with anyone, but I've had sex with two people in the last whatever." And I said, "Cute." He's like, "I've only slept with you." I'm like, "Well, that's nice, *but* . . . " Anyway, so we went on talking about it.

DL: This was when?

Sebastian: This was my first semester coming back after England. And after being on and off in the relationship. And obviously knowing that he had, you know, we'd be seeing other people but I knew, I still assumed that he would tell me if he'd been with someone else. And so we talked about this for a long time, then he had to go to work. I already made him late—45 minutes late. That was the other thing I said. I said, "If I didn't find this, how would I know?" The other thing I said is, "I know a maid comes all the time. How recent did this happen? And that you were with someone like right before you were with me?" You know, that I also got . . . I don't know, it bothered me. That's my own personal preference, whatever. And so that was the whole situation. He then explained that the maid hadn't come for about 2 weeks but I still was, 2 weeks is still too soon for me. Anyways, a couple weeks later I finally . . . And first of all I told him right there, I said, "Whoof, our sexual relationship has just ended. Right there." And he was like, "well what about our friendship" and everything else, and blah blah blah, and I said, "I have to think about that." And that's how I left it. And I flew back up here. And came back up here. Told him um . . . finally talked to him about 2 weeks later, I called him up and said we have to talk about this. And he's like, "Okay." He's like, "I'm glad you called." I said, "first of all . . . " Well I started to talk about it and I told him how upset I was and that he didn't tell me this and that I felt betrayed and stuff and he's like well maybe we just didn't understand each other's communications and stuff, he gave me that, and I said, "Stop right there. Who cares what. . . . Forget whatever communication we had or whatever agreement we had. Don't you think in this day and age that you owe it to someone to tell them before you engage in anything that's unsafe?"

DL: I guess he felt he'd been safe, huh?

Sebastian: He felt he'd been safe. And I said, don't you owe it to him to tell him? Even an occurrence that you may think is safe? I mean, you know about this, too. I said, irrelevant of anything we may have decided as a person and as someone who knows, you should tell me.

DL: And especially he'd had unsafe sex with you and how could he know for sure what you had done?

Sebastian: Mm-hm.

DL: I guess.

Sebastian: And I told him that, and he, he agreed with me, I mean, he had to agree. I think he was shocked you know, that I said, that I didn't just go well, you promised me. I was like, irrelevant. Irrelevant of all that, you owed it to me, as a person. You know, period. And if you don't have that type of belief, I mean, just forget it right there.

Sebastian was lucky enough to learn the lesson without any physical harm. Nor were women completely immune from this type of thinking, though Ann was the only woman who expressed it: "I didn't suspect that any of my partners had [injected drugs] because most of them were pretty straight, clean."

DIFFICULTY OF NEGOTIATING SAFE SEX

Even for those who had managed to incorporate some safer-sex practice into their relationships, it wasn't always easy. Only Hanan expressed no ambivalence about insisting on condom use. Denise felt she was doing the best she could:

Even though I am up front and they need a condom, it's still, I mean I'm not saying that that's not hard for me to do, too, like if you're in the moment, I'm not saying that oh yeah, I'm so together that it's just really easy for me to grab it, I mean it takes extra, I mean it really takes some extra pressure from yourself to say "Go get the condom," you know, I mean, I'm, I'm not saying that it's easy for me to just be able to do that, but I know there is that extra little thing in me that says go get the condom, that's it. But now for me to be able to say go get the condom and the foam and everything else, it might be, that might be a little bit harder for me than just having the condom ready.

However, she resented having to be always in charge:

It seems like I'm gonna be taking all the steps one step at a time, and most men don't seem to be taking the same steps that I'm taking, is kind of how it feels sometimes, too. I mean, not that that should deter me, but it just seems like such a lopsided issue sometimes, the whole idea of protection.

When Janice tried to refuse sex with her boyfriend, he behaved

like he's wounded. "What, you don't like me? Oh no, what do you
mean?" . . . And instead of me communicating then what was going
on, I didn't. So it snowballed and every time he said let's have sex, by
me having sex it was like proving to him that I still liked him.

Marianna found it easier to ask for what she wanted with partners
she didn't care about very much. However, even she found it difficult
to insist on safe sex, finding situations more ambiguous in the moment.

DL: So with Jack, how did you talk about it with Jack? How did it come
up with him?

Marianna: Um . . . He was a real fetishist, so we had to talk about it anyway, things that he liked, so him bringing up things that he liked or
wanted me to try to do. It was a lot easier for me to say okay then I
want to do this and that, this and that.

DL: 'Cause he was making himself vulnerable first?

Marianna: Um, yeah, uh, and I'm not sure if vulnerable's the right word,
I know that he doesn't care at all, like, that—that . . . So that was a
big experience. And then . . .

DL: So did you talk about safe sex with him? Specifically? Rather than
just what you want to do in bed?

Marianna: Um . . . I think only so far as if you're gonna be inside me there
has to be latex, but . . . But even that didn't happen once, you know,
so it . . . We talked about it but I wasn't really adamant about enforc-
ing it.

DL: Why not, do you think?

Marianna: I don't know. It . . . [long pause] Maybe sometimes I just expect
people to do what they say they're gonna do. You know? And all of
a sudden you're in it and you're wait, whoa, but you're already in it.

DL: What do you imagine about your next relationship?

Marianna: I don't know. Total unknown. . . . I think I'm looking for a girl
date but I don't know . . . Yeah. And I don't know about safe sex
within this next relationship. I really don't feel like I know what I'm
doing.

DL: About safe sex?

Marianna: Yeah. About *doing* it. You know? It's not about what you're
supposed to do, but *how* to do that. How to do that when you're really
in bed. It's really hard.

Negotiating for safer sex contained elements of impression management, required assertiveness, and took constant effort, even for those who had made the most progress in incorporating it.

GUYS DON'T FEEL RISK

I heard repeatedly from both men and women that men didn't question their partners about their sexual histories. There seemed to be a consensus among women that men didn't think about risk, "It's like guys don't even care so they, like even the guy that I slept with who I don't even know his name" (Denise). Ann was rather nonchalant about men's nature:

> Ann: Guys don't worry about those things.
>
> DL: Why, do you think? What makes you think that, and then why do you think that?
>
> Ann: They're *guys*. 'Cause I think guys are much more right in the here and now, and so they're just more interested in scoring than having the discussion that could get in the way or something. I don't think they're as concerned and I think maybe at some point afterwards every now and then they'll maybe think about it but I think guys are just less worried about what's happening later on.
>
> DL: So they don't feel risk?
>
> Ann: Yeah, maybe, it's just sort of like they're doing what they're doing and it's so abstract to think that 10 years from now they might get sick 'cause you're jumping into bed with somebody right now. So I think that guys don't, they're not as cautious, or they're not as concerned and I think for the most part they don't like using condoms anyways so they don't really want to. So if they could get away with not doing it they'd just as soon not. And it's only, it's like with just birth control in general it always falls on the female's responsibility because, unless the female actually says anything I, I couldn't even imagine any of the guys I know taking the initiative.

Janice was having a harder time with her partner's resistance to condoms:

> Whereas Rob doesn't think that . . . or he would say things like, "Can I just put it in for a minute?" And my girlfriend got pregnant like that. So, I think "what is your problem?" It's like sometimes he's a 15 year old who just got an erection and he doesn't know what to do with it. . . . That's really what's been affecting me, looking at this relationship going, you know, there's a lot more going on than just your penis.

Rita's impression differed from that of other women; she thought the men she knew *were* concerned about risk,

> I know a lot of guys are scared about AIDS. Just from my perception and from our discussion, we were talking. The guys did mention, "Oh, well, STDs and AIDS. I'd want to be safe. I'd want to know if that girl had some sort of disease or virus or something because that would be unfair for me not to know."

As Ann understood, it wasn't that men didn't think about risk. For men who proceed with intercourse without using condoms, it might just be after the fact.

> DL: That was the first time in your life that it happened?
>
> Donald: Yeah. That I've had sex without a condom. And that was last semester. First and only time. So.
>
> DL: So did that make you worried for yourself?
>
> Donald: Afterwards it did, during, no

> Joseph: I think he assumed I was no risk, and I didn't think about it with him, I guess, as far as asking him if he was at risk. We talked about it later, he said he's slept with one guy and that's it. Now I wonder if that's true or not, I've talked to other people and they've made certain comments. But I, I wonder. I've been meaning to ask him again.

> Shawn: I was worried about her, you know, getting pregnant but I was also 10 times, you know, a thousand times more worried about just like getting AIDS from her, you know, I was just, I'm ascared of it, it scares the hell out of me.

> George: The interesting thing is, it wasn't brought up until we were actually having intercourse, and it was at that moment right when we were having intercourse that we looked at each other, both of us at the same time and said what are we doing?

It appeared that although they worried about exposure to an STD, men tended to rely more on information such as partner's background and lifestyle than on actual questioning about sexual history.

SAFER-SEX TALK

Talking about safer sex, discussing a prospective partner's history, is not something that comes easily or that young people are trained to do. How easily the conversation occurs depends partly on the status of the relationship and partly on how easily each person can acknowledge that his or her intention is sexual.

When Sebastian had sex with a neighbor on summer vacations, neither partner was "out," making discussion about what they were doing impossible. Such reticence was not exclusive to gay relationships, because the dynamics are not dissimilar for many young people beginning to be sexual. Unfortunately, safer-sex discussions are more often than not limited to recounting how many partners one has had. Trust was thus initially constructed by evaluating a potential partner's previous relationship patterns. Most often the subject was broached indirectly:

> Donald: We just talked about [it] even more casually, it was more just general conversations about who we've been with or who—and it wasn't like I was probing or she was probing, it was just we were talking and it came out, somebody she'd slept—you know, somebody she knew or somebody she'd been with, and just who she's been involved with over the years.

With Karen it was a little more direct. "We talked about her, and then who else he had been seeing at Berkeley and he told me and then he told how many people he had sex with and I told him and one night we just talked about it." Ginger would "bluntly" ask her partners how many partners they'd had, when they last got out of a relationship, the nature of the relationship, the extent of their emotional involvement, whether it had been long term or a one-night stand.

Although George repeatedly stressed the importance of communication, the fact that he did begin intercourse without communication illustrates some dissonance between his attitudes and his behavior. He continued telling me about the incident:

> DL: So after you've already started.
>
> George: Yeah, after we've already started and then we sat back and starting talking.
>
> DL: So what did you do, you'd already started, it went through both your minds, what happened next?
>
> George: We stopped and we started talking about it and I said, "We need to talk about what's going on" and she said, "Well I don't really feel like I want to talk about it now." I said, "Well you know, that we shouldn't be doing that if we can't talk about things, because it's not healthy."

DL: Uh huh. And what did she say?

George: She gave me a big hug and she didn't express herself in words but she gave me a big hug and you know, it was a comfortable hug like you know, wow, I'm glad that you can stop and be able to talk to me about this rather than just being selfish. . . . I think that it's really important, that it's not talked about and it's started, you need to stop right away and before anything else happens you need to talk about it and so we talked about it, and we felt comfortable and the amazing thing is, and I wish people could realize once you talk about it, and you know what's going on and you know what this person is, it's just not the physical aspects of what sex offers, but you got to look at somebody and trust them and it makes things so much more comfortable and the mental feeling of what sex is really about. . . .

They "talked about it," but because neither had ever been tested for any STDs, they didn't really have evidence for the confidence George displayed.

George: I found out at the moment that she was on the pill. Okay, so we had basically said this is what our sexual histories are, I don't think that I've ever had anything, you don't think you have anything, okay that's fine. But we haven't come into a situation where we've been sexually active since then, so it really hasn't come up. I mean if we go out and we do something, and we go and have lunch or something, it's not like we're just going to say, "oh, by the way, you know, what happens the next time we do it?" I think we're going to wait until the next time it happens.

DL: And then?

George: And then figure out what we want to do. We basically already know each other's histories and where we're coming from, so I think that the hardest part is out. Now, whether or not she knows, we know that she's on the pill, whether or not she wants me to use a condom is fine, I mean I won't feel offended. I won't feel anything at all. It's not like it matters to me.

George didn't see any need to protect himself and didn't intend to use a condom unless his partner requested it. Vicky found herself in a similar situation (it almost sounded like the same encounter) but handled it slightly differently:

Like when we went there . . . I mean I got drunk I mean I was under the influence but I had enough control to stop it so I know that it wasn't just under . . . it was because I wanted it too. So you know we were out on the balcony and we started kissing and we just came into the room and . . . this is where it stopped. I stopped him, like, he—he actually stopped—no, okay, we were getting a little passionate there and I said, and I said, "Are you gonna use anything?" I asked him, and he goes, "Yeah, of course, I am." And he got up and he went into his room and got a condom and everything and um, he came into the room and it was funny because he goes, "See" and he showed me and I thought that was, you know, kind of funny and then we just you know started kissing again and I pushed him off me and—this is where I'll think you'll find it interesting—we were sitting there like pretty much butt naked, sitting there and we started . . . and I said, "You know . . ."—actually this is very embarrassing. He's in my class that you came into, so I stopped and I said, "What did we learn in class?" See, having him in my class, it was a lot easier to talk about this because that was the topic of discussion and you know, we were sitting there, I said, you know, "Hey, what did we talk about in class?" First of all, with him, I could be open and second of all, because he was in my class, it was so much easier because we were talking about this and how important it was and I said, "What did we talk about in class?" He goes, he goes, he goes . . . he didn't say, "Are you kidding?" or anything. He was serious too and he goes, he goes, "Well, I'm using a condom" and he was, you know, "we talked about that in class." "What other girls have you been with, I don't even know." So we were sitting there talking about it you know, like he told me he was with three other girls, he used condoms da da da and I was sitting there. And he goes, "Well what about you?" you know, and this and that . . .

Dave had difficulty talking about sexual histories with his partner:

I tried to ask him about the history of his sexual partners, like asking him if he had—I can't remember exactly what I said, but something related to just finding out how many boyfriends, or how many people he had sex with kinda thing. And he would not, he didn't really want to discuss about it. He told me that he didn't, he—quote—like "I don't want to talk about my history."

Dave wasn't too worried about it, though, because they hadn't engaged in anal sex. He would indicate that he wasn't comfortable performing or receiving what he considered a risky act by saying it didn't turn him on, for him a safer-sex strategy.

Andrew's safer-sex discussion with his girlfriend led to an argument. When he told her his history in the initial stages of the relationship, she didn't say anything about herself, so he assumed that she had also always practiced safe sex. He learned a year later that she'd been mostly unsafe with her previous partner, who was

> a fly-by-night, a sketchy guy, a businessman, and then he had all kinds of different partners, things like that, but it was just that I told her right away and she told me that she assumed that I knew that she meant she had unprotected sex by her silence, which was ridiculous, and she knew that too.

Where the risk is felt more personally or the sex is unusual, safer sex is easier to talk about. Marianna had had the most varied experience of all the participants in terms of numbers of partners and range of practice and definitely had safer sex on her mind. A ménage à trois had raised some issues for her with

> a heterosexual couple. And a couple of people. And they um, . . . they'd been together 2½ or 3 years at that point and she'd just gone on the pill, and I don't know if they were using latex before or not but anyway, that her going on the pill definitely was, you know, part of not having to deal with anything but each other now. And I found myself thinking things like, "Okay, well can I kiss her now?" Or like, I wasn't sexually involved with them enough that I had to bring up latex. And they weren't um, but it was really interesting the list of things that started happening in my mind. It's like if we're ever gonna do this again we have to talk about all these things. Like, you know, I have to list all these things that I—'cause they're obviously not thinking about me in relation to it at all.

Janice felt that sex with a bisexual man would relieve her of the responsibility of broaching safer sex. Instead of *whether* to practice safer sex, as with Rob, the issue with Andre would be *how:*

> DL: So if you decide to let him initiate, how would you take care of yourself as far as contraceptives? Or as far as safe sex?
>
> Janice: Well, that's another thing that's really interesting because I would have to because he's 29. He's a bisexual which I don't have a problem with in general but then, when specifically, when I think of him that I know he's been a slut in the past and he's talked about it. Since we work in a health clinic together and we've had classes, and I mean they've been pretty serious and in depth. And they've been about sexually transmitted diseases he's mentioned a couple and one thing he mentioned was genital warts. And that's one thing that I just don't want to have anything to do with. And I have talked to him about

that too that I was afraid of getting involved with anyone, and I didn't mean him. But he just said that, no, you just have to have a lot of safe sex. But see part of me doesn't trust men who say that, because my boyfriend now will say, because we're always in between whether I'm using the pill or the diaphragm or just using condoms. He's got it in his head that I could sort of like predict my ovulation. And that if I knew this were day 15 that it would be okay. So that if I were on my period then everything would be okay, which might make sense, but then a week after my period doesn't make sense as much. But he would sort of say, "Well is it still okay, can we have sex without a condom?" And that's when all this problem with him started because I thought, "What is he doing?" He's not respecting what I'm doing. He's thinking about sex as if it's good for him but he's not thinking about how different it is for me who's got to think about, wait a minute, this is something serious. And I don't want to get pregnant and I don't want to deal with pregnancy. 'Cause luckily with Rob, that's all we've had to worry about is pregnancy.

TRUST AND SEX

Several participants mentioned that a certain level of trust would be needed to engage in specific sex acts. Denise generally refused oral sex with men but not women, "Yeah although they would like to. To me oral sex too is more intimate, I don't know why. But to me oral sex is more—I don't know why—intimate than actual sex." (I wondered what she thought "actual sex" would be with a woman.) Starting with a casual encounter, Dave gauged he was in love after a month, because "I've sort of said to myself that I won't really engage in receiving anal sex until I'm ready for a relationship. And it has to be someone special. So I did it." Hanan mostly thought fellatio wasn't safe enough:

I don't go down on people. I don't give oral sex. I have once, but the person I had been with was the same person I had first slept with so I had known him for 8 years. He had been tested for AIDS every 6 months, so I knew.

Marianna felt similarly about intercourse with a man:

There was one time once with someone that I really, really trust a lot where he entered me without a condom, and I said, "What are you doing?" And he entered me and came out and he's like "that was it, I'm sorry." Really. But it didn't affect my trust and it didn't affect the

sex. Which is different, really different. I feel really differently about
him than I've felt about guys in a long time.

It follows, then, that if one engages too easily in sexual behavior that
is considered intimate, one becomes suspect. Vicky used condoms
with her partner because of the reputation of one of his previous
partners:

> Vicky: Yeah because my current boyfriend now—the one I'm not talking
> to now, I don't know what our status is. He went out with this girl
> who was known to be pretty promiscuous, like you know, she was
> known to give good head, she was known to um, . . .
>
> DL: Do you have to be promiscuous to give good head?
>
> Vicky: No. [laughs] I mean she was known to be promiscuous, like you
> know, "oh, she gives good head" and they would talk about her and
> you know, certain things you would know like someone is very ac-
> tive, I guess what I'm saying. They, you know, my girlfriends call her
> a 'ho and the whole bit you know and she does this and that. She's
> really nasty, she'll do every position with you and she'll do it with
> you the first night and just the whole thing. Anyway, he went out
> with her and I mean that worries me a lot that he went out with her.

The Construction of Risk

Most of the participants had fairly accurate information about
transmission of HIV. They made decisions about specific sexual acts
within the context of the type of relationship in which they were
involved. For example, most students accepted condoms for genital
or anal intercourse as a fact of modern sexual life. Among those who
practiced fellatio, they had decided that oral sex without ejaculation
was an acceptable risk. Protecting themselves from other STDs had
occurred only to Andrew, not arising as an issue even among those
who had previously contracted an STD. The gay men were certainly
most aware of the reality of risk for HIV, but there were no other
defining characteristics that predicted how seriously an individual
would take HIV.

For Andrew, it was his future orientation that made him take risk
seriously.

> DL: Why do you suppose you take the risk seriously when other people
> your age don't?

Andrew: I don't know. I paid attention in Social Living in high school. [laughs] When I was 15 actually I got picked from my school to sit with a panel of people to talk about, at Cal, to tell these teachers about how to teach AIDS to kids. And I had no training or anything, one of the teachers just liked the way I talked about it when I was younger and so they threw me up on this panel on campus and it was kind of cool. I really, it just scares me. I think it's like—I think, you know what it might be also that I thought, I'm working on a lot of things right now in my life. I'm trying to do all these different things, I'm putting a lot of investment into my life. I'm taking time to sit in classrooms and listen to self-important teachers tell me what they think is okay. And I am writing and I am reading and I am doing all these new things. And that's why I have an investment in something. And I am thinking, "Do you want to ruin that for something like . . . ?" You know, because I thought, I mean I always imagined what it would be like if you got the diagnosis of AIDS. How stupid would you feel? If you got it getting it from, if you knew you got it from sexual contact. Where you could have just reached over and grabbed a condom and that's why the thing when they said that, that report came out, you know how the media jumps on those things, they said, "The condom might not be all that great at protecting you from AIDS." I saw it and I thought, "Great. That's just what people need to hear. Now they are not going to use them even more." But I don't want to be one of those nights when they are talking on TV, and they say, "Do you use condoms when you have sex?" "Nope." "Why not?" "'Cause I have natural, heterosexual sex, and I don't need them."

According to Dave, who volunteered at the Free Clinic, oral sex without using condoms was safe enough, even though intellectually he knew differently:

DL: So would you do it without the condom then?

Dave: Yeah. I think to a certain extent that is actually quite common from what I hear in the gay community.

DL: To have oral sex without condoms?

Dave: Not so much to the point of ejaculation, but just um, sucking without condoms.

DL: And then do you stop before ejaculation?

Dave: Yeah.

DL: What about pre-ejaculate? It's sort of like an acceptable risk?

Dave: Yeah . . . I think I know the risks and you know when clients come in I do tell them that there is a possibility of transmission.

DL: So it . . . How do you work it out in your mind?

Dave: In . . .

DL: Acceptable risk?

Dave: I think I know the risks. It's like . . . I mean I wouldn't go out and perform oral sex if I'm having sores or something or my gum is bleeding, so I think that greatly reduces um . . .

It was interesting that in the midst of discussing his *personal* risk behavior, he switched to the third person counselor-client role. Creating distance this way to make the notion of personal risk less threatening was not unusual. Shawn visualized a discussion between two internal selves:

Shawn: I was just . . . at that moment and we were both there and she just kinda slipped it in and I wasn't really in the point to kind of hold back, I was just like—and right when I was in—and then when I was inside, I mean, when I was in her, I was just sitting there going, I was just like—I was in so much like mental ecstasy there, it was so . . . And then, on the other hand, it's kinda like that little TV show where all those guys are up there controlling the brain, like one's of 'em's just going "YEAH! YEAH!" and the other one is going—the con person's going "NO! NO!" and that's exactly . . .

DL: So was there somebody going, "God, I hope she doesn't have anything"?

Shawn: Oh! Yeah! Oh! *Definitely!* I mean, right—I mean like the other person up there's just going "Okay"—like the logical and analytical person's up there goin' "Okay, she comes from a good, she lives in a good house, she comes from a good family, she has a lot of social grace, you know, but going through a just like oh pleasepleaseplease I hope she has nothing—or anything." And then, he's also sitting up there going "Okay this is it, do it really quickly you know so less chance, you know, less time in there, you know, maybe you know that'll make sure that there's no, you know, less chance of catching something."

TRANSMISSION INFORMATION AND SAFER SEX

If risk then is assessed in terms of mutual trust and degree of intimacy in the relationship, it is applied only to the extent that accurate information about transmission is known, believed, *and* personalized. Ann and George, particularly, held information that they manipulated to rationalize their risk behavior and explain why safer sex was not necessary for them. It didn't occur to George somehow that his partner could transmit an STD and not know about it, even though he knew differently intellectually.

DL: You didn't get around to telling me how—I asked how you came to decide what you guys should use and what was important? You said that neither of you had been tested for AIDS?

George: Yeah.

DL: You didn't say if you've been tested for any other STDs?

George: I haven't. But with the facts that I have been presented with, if I were to have a commonly known STD, I would have probably found out by now. Whether it's chlamydia, or gonorrhea, even though men don't show that many symptoms for chlamydia, I would think that from my previous sexual history I would have probably, it would have probably come up by now.

DL: How's that?

George: Umm . . . Visually, physically, and one of the reasons I think that way is because my brother contracted an STD and he found out and he knew like 2 days after he'd been with this person that he had. And so that's always been stuck in my mind, 'cause he's my brother, and I think the people you are close with, it sticks. And he found out a couple days afterwards, and so that's just kind of how I think I don't have anything. Now whether or not—and second of all, I don't think it's healthy to go and get paranoid about everything that's out there, I think in our society we've taken it to such an extreme with AIDS that we're so fearful of AIDS, the word AIDS and I don't think that it's healthy, I just don't. I don't think that every time you have sex with somebody, you should go and you should have to be tested, if you take the preventative measures you know, beforehand that you shouldn't . . .

DL: So what kind of preventative measures did you take with this partner?

George: We talked about it. We talked about our previous sexual histories and she had basically said well this is who I'd been with, and these are the men that I've slept with, and this is—I haven't had anything noticeable, and I basically said the same thing, and so we felt comfortable, which I think is *fine*. It might not be the moralistic thing to do, but, the bottom line is that we talked about it, whether the trust is at a hundred percent, I don't know, in all honesty, I don't know how she lives her life, I don't know if she's lying to me, but I trust her, and the same thing goes, she doesn't know if I'm lying to her about any of those things, she doesn't know if I'm a compulsive male or that I have HIV or that I go sleeping around with people just to get people HIV, you don't know that.

DL: Right.

George: And I think that you *should* know that because it makes things really uncomfortable. I think in the most idealistic relationship, yes, you've gotta sit down with someone across the table and you need to say, okay you tell me about everything that you've ever done, and I want to know all the times you had sex, and all the unprotected times, and, oh for that one time that you didn't use a condom, well maybe you should go get tested. I don't think that that's, I mean, I think, that's idealistic but it's not realistic. Because we treat sex as a taboo subject, it's such a taboo subject in the society where it's not within the relationships yet, just being able to sit across from somebody and explain to somebody sex, and what you've done, and where you're coming from, and who you've slept with, and all the experiences that you've ever had.

George's construction didn't have a great deal of room in it for people contracting STDs without being aware of it. Ann created distance by separating herself from the kind of woman she considered *really* at risk (i.e., "the female equivalent of Wilt Chamberlain.") She had a clever metaphor ready to counter any argument I proposed.

DL: Even after the first time [did you say], "Okay we kind of blew it last night. Let's talk about this"?

Ann: Yeah, well, then you've got the theory that what's done is done and so what's the use now, kind of thing which is I know also not too realistic because maybe last night we were lucky or whatever but still we can make up for that. Like I said before, it seems if, if you're gonna use condoms or whatever, you really should use them all the time and so maybe that's just an excuse so that the one time after you don't use it, that you decide not to again just to scrap the whole idea or something.

DL: The analogy that strikes me then is the diet analogy. You know, just 'cause you blow it and have an ice cream sundae one night, does that mean you blow the whole diet?

Ann: Well, that, I wouldn't really liken it to that because . . . eat, eating an ice cream sundae, you could still lose that weight but if you contracted a virus, you can't un-contract it by being good after that.

DL: What if there's um—people don't know everything about AIDS yet and what if there's a, it takes a certain amount of exposure—to be exposed 10 times, you don't necessarily contract it the first time the virus gets into your system, but you need, but if you're exposed 10 times, you have more chance.

Ann: Then you hope you're not sleeping with somebody 10 times that has the virus?

DL: But what I mean is, so if you blow it one time . . . ?

Ann: Right. Then, um, I don't know, I hadn't ever thought of it in that theory and the disease contraction thing. My roommate, her gyne-cologist told her something like even if you slept with somebody and had unprotected sex with somebody who had the virus, you still had a 1 in 500 chance of getting it or something like that. I don't know, I think that was pretty irresponsible because after hearing that, it was just of like, "Whoa, then forget about it. Who needs safe sex, 1 in 500," like you said, everybody chooses where, it's like (a) what's the prob-ability that my boyfriend is HIV positive? and (b) even if he was, you know . . .

DL: Well, if he were HIV positive, isn't there a possibility that you could have sex 500 times in the course of a relationship?

Ann: Yeah, but by then I would have found out he was HIV positive.

DL: . . . And then what would you do?

Ann: [laughs] Be really upset. I'd sue him. That's what all Americans do. I'd go to court, I'd get a lawyer and—no, I'm sure that I would prob-ably, no, I'm sure I would not sleep with him anymore. I'd be really upset and probably fanatically test myself for the next however much time until I felt secure about that. And also probably be so, so disen-chanted with men from him lying to me that I'd, I'd never want to go out with another one again and I'd be very distrustful, so I'd have to join some man-hater's club.

George distinguished risk between pregnancy and STDs. Like Ann, he could separate himself from those he considered truly risky.

Well, obviously, my opinion is unsafe sex is somebody who you just meet, you don't talk about things and you don't use any kind of con-traception, birth control or prevention against STDs. Okay, the girl that I'm seeing right now, we practice safe sex for contraception. She's on the birth control pill and that's all that we practice. Whether or not, whether or not, you know, we have never been tested for HIV. Previous to the sexual experiences . . . But I think that we communicate, we feel that trust that if—I don't know, there's always that risk, you know if we haven't been tested, she hasn't been tested, I haven't been tested, there's no way that we would know. There's an outside chance that yeah, wow, I could be HIV positive but that's not just something that I've incorporated in things that would happen to me.

George and Ann were particularly frustrating to listen to because they were obviously bright, knew the facts, but had somehow been able to deny the connection between their behavior and risk.

At the time of our interview, Raphael held an inaccurate idea of transmission that might have proved dangerous:

DL: How many times had you been together before you decided that each other were safe?

Raphael: Gosh. [pause] Probably a couple weeks, 2 or 3 weeks. I don't really remember.

DL: Did you have intercourse without a condom?

Raphael: We have once, but we don't usually. I mean I'm always doer, usually, I mean, except for once, and then we didn't . . . complete the act, I guess.

DL: So what happened that one time that you didn't have one?

Raphael: Well usually whenever we have sex it's always him usually asking for it, 'cause I guess he's into anal stimulation, and so usually we've used one, a condom every time except for once. And I think we had been drinking, you know, it's like we had gone into a club and all of a sudden it's let's go and we had been drinking. I probably had thought of using one but knowing that I had just been tested and I hadn't been with anybody else, it didn't really bother me that much.

KNOWLEDGE INTO ACTION

Even when risk was felt and acted on, it was still difficult to take all the precautions that might have been considered necessary. Denise wasn't the only one who had difficulty with the "extra pressure" of having safer sex. Marianna described the difficulty of assessing risk and following through in her sexual relationships.

DL: You don't feel like you're a risk, it sounds like. Do you feel like you're a risk to somebody else?

Marianna: No, but see that's still not a good enough reason to not do it [practice safer sex], you know. No, I don't feel like I'm risky. But in my brain that's, that doesn't necessarily equal—although that's probably the bottom line reason you're not insisting 'cause you're not scared, and they're not, it sounds like a lot of people aren't scared. A lot of guys aren't scared.

DL: Why is that, do you think?

Marianna: It doesn't have anything to do with them. You know, they like girls, you know? And I think there's also even still, and even among younger people, that whole thing, um . . . you know, if you get sick from sex you could fix it? You know, it's easy to fix. And that even though it's not true they think that's the way.

DL: Has anybody ever asked you if you've been tested for anything?

Marianna: Yeah, it comes up.

DL: How does that come up?

Marianna: They'll just, you know, "Have you been tested, how was it?" But, you know, that doesn't mean shit. I mean most people who know me well know that I'm honest, but, I mean that doesn't mean shit when you don't know somebody well, you know, you don't know nothing about them that way.

Like the women in Kemp's study (1993), she and her partner epitomized the attitude of many women who feel that lesbian sex is safe, even if the partners are not monogamous—or not lesbians.

DL: Did you, if you felt at risk enough to get yourself tested, when you went back with Linda, did you take any special precautions then?

Marianna: No, no. I didn't. We've *never* practiced safe sex. She and I have not.

DL: What would make you think you needed to?

Marianna: Some of it was that you, I felt that I should learn how with someone that I really care about, like the best, it's really, first sexual encounters are hard enough without learning how to do something new, um, but that logic didn't go over real well with her.

DL: You mean you brought it up?

Marianna: Yeah. We talked about it. She was really mad at me. I mean she's been really mad at me, sometimes I think she's been overreacting and sometimes totally rightfully so. Um, there's her stuff . . .

DL: How did the discussion go when you brought it up? What did you say and what did she say?

Marianna: I'm not sure I remember. I um I'm sure I brought it up as far as us trying to see what it was like to be totally safe.

Her partner broke up with her because she'd had sex (using a condom) with a man. Marianna found it ironic:

Marianna: Um, she moved out. And yeah, that was actually a big one. That was a very big one because that's when I found out that she was using our dildo with Julie and not—not only without latex, but without sterilizing it. And it's like—I'm busted for safe sex and you're worried about with Julie? Hel*lo*.

DL: So it was going on on both sides.

Marianna: Yeah, except it doesn't count on her side. To her it still doesn't count.

DL: Why?

Marianna: Um . . . 'Cause girls were safe. And I can't, you know, I can say it and she can say it, but it's not as bad. And there's nothing I can say. No, it's not as bad—*but* . . . .

Wheeler also felt that trust couldn't be constructed by recounting sexual histories, that only behavior made one accountable.

DL: Does anybody ever ask you, have partners asked you if you've been tested?

Wheeler: Not a one. I volunteer the information but no one has ever asked me.

DL: Are you surprised?

Wheeler: Yeah. Then again, I haven't asked either.

DL: Do you have some way of checking out a partner's history? Do you get them to tell you their story?

Wheeler: You know . . . I guess I don't see the relevance of it. Because you can contract HIV if you've had one partner or if you've had 500. . . . And for me safer sex is safer sex and if I'm practicing safer sex then . . . people can lie, people can be genuinely misinformed if they could have contracted it in the past 6 months, so if I ask you if you are positive or negative, with the intent that we're going to go to bed afterwards, if you tell me yes or no, I still don't have any way of knowing.

In spite of all the available information, safer sex is incorporated incrementally as individuals attend to the messages and apply them to themselves. Even then, they discriminate among partners, behaviors, and levels of risk in ways that are sometimes not congruent with the accepted biomedical reality of the time.

6

Negotiating Sex

The overarching struggle between risk and trust in relationships remains the difficulty of attaining a balance between protecting oneself by assuming one's partner poses some risk and believing that the partner is trustworthy. Trust is demonstrated by using methods that are unequivocally oriented to contraception and not STD protection, presenting a conflict between pregnancy prevention and safer sex. Both men and women spoke of the need to behave, first, as though sex were not planned and second, as though the relationship were serious when still in its early stages. Furthermore, though condom use was the main strategy for reducing risk, not everyone felt comfortable negotiating it. Other general strategies included minimizing exposure to semen and testing for HIV antibodies to ascertain partners' serostatus.

Condoms, Dental Dams, and Spermicide

CONDOMS, CONTRACEPTION, AND SAFER SEX

Grimley et al. (1993) and Maticka-Tyndale (1991a, 1991b, p. 45) and others have suggested that contraceptive use follows a developmental pattern beginning with no method, incorporating condoms, and last, beginning the use of oral contraceptives. In the first 3 weeks of their relationship, Charlie and his girlfriend used no contraception. They decided that he should buy some, but he was embarrassed about what the pharmacist might think. Later, he learned to take responsibility for maintaining adequate supplies, considering it his due because she had to worry about risk. Sonia preferred to stock the condoms herself so she wouldn't have to worry. Vicky liked condoms because they were the easiest. Sarita said she "would just tell myself that as long as the condom was put on before it got hot and heavy let's say that it would be okay and I couldn't get pregnant. And that's all I was worried about was getting pregnant." Mary made her partner stop to put on a condom during intercourse her first time, even though she thought it might be "pointless" by then. Andrew felt that it had been acceptable to put on a condom for contraception part way through because he wasn't worried about contracting an STD from his steady partner.

Dave used two condoms and lubricant for anal sex. Wheeler also used a condom for anal sex, with the understanding that a new partner would have the same expectations as he.

> When we were having sex, at the point at which I felt that we needed to use a condom, it was kind of a mutual thing. He knew that it was necessary, I knew that it was necessary, and I said, "Okay, well, it's time to get out some protection," when we were going to engage in anal sex. So it wasn't something we discussed necessarily beforehand, but when it came up in the heat of the moment it was an expectation on both our parts.

However, with a different partner, "there was one time when his expectation was different from mine and he didn't want to use a condom, and I did and there was a little tug of war there but not much because I was very firm." Still, Wheeler and some of the others had consented to unprotected sex using withdrawal, as the

> one night we were making love and we didn't have a condom and we went to a certain point and then we stopped . . . just because it kind of scared me. So I said, "Okay we need to stop, I don't feel comfortable with this." And he was supportive of that.

ACCEPTING THE NOTION OF RISK

Although they might not feel open about discussing condoms before a sexual encounter, several participants felt strongly that they would not engage in intercourse without a condom. In Sebastian's only sexual encounter with a woman, she had planned the seduction in advance, with the condom ready:

> She had it. Which was good. I mean I wasn't gonna go that far, I mean, it was, if that was the case, I knew after being at Berkeley for that time I had known, learned enough about safe sex and was interested in it, and—not even interested, it was a believer in it and not going to partake in it without in relation to women at that time. Um . . . And so you know, I knew we needed a condom, she had one. She'd actually come to my, I was out the night before and she'd come and she'd bought it, she said, "You know where I bought this?" I'm like, "No, where?" "I bought it downstairs in the bathroom at your place when I came to visit you."

Karen had had an encounter with a new partner before he learned he'd been exposed to an STD; she'd also developed a bladder infection as a result of beginning the new relationship. Even though she was conscientiously taking the pill, they added condoms after the unprotected encounter because they "decided that that was pretty stupid and so we did every time after that for it's been 6 months." Andrew had also adapted:

> I actually have psyched myself out about it. I'll do the old "1 in 250. You may not get AIDS but you could get something else really nasty. Not all STDs are curable. Even if they are, they are not that fun." And so I just was like, "save yourself the anguish and take 2 seconds."

He found that he really didn't mind them:

> The only disadvantage is that you have to go "Urr, wait" and then put it on and, otherwise, the feeling and all that, I can live with that. I really have not thought, "This sucks, man, this sucks." I think if you have them near the bed, or something like that, and you can just go whoosh, I mean what does it take? Five or ten seconds if you know what you are doing, and it really is not that bad a thing to me.

Jacob had trained himself similarly:

> I've heard everybody say, "Oh, it takes something off the romance, you have to stop." And even though from time to time I'll feel god, I have to stop and have to get out the condom and have to put it on, but I guess it's become so routine it's something I need to do.

He didn't envision being able to forego condoms even in a monogamous long-term relationship, because "there would be that doubt. I
mean that slight chance because you can't be certain about anything.
Especially when it comes to HIV." Lauren and her friends would now
interrupt a sexual encounter to find a condom to keep themselves
safe, and in fact, one participant left a woman's apartment in the
middle of the night to fetch a condom. Andrew had refused women
who told him "Don't worry about it." His response was, "No, you're
crazy. I'm not going to do that."

RESISTANCE TO CONDOMS

Hanan, who said she had never had intercourse without a condom, expressed the importance of safe sex thus: "Strap it or wrap it
or do whatever you have to do. I'm not goin' down with anybody."
Hanan was confident that "if someone has a problem with it that's a
personal problem, it's not mine, and I will take myself out of the
situation." After Sonia had gotten pregnant, she insisted on condoms.
When her partner (later husband) complained, she refused to have
sex with him for 6 or 7 months. Denise was interested in a sexual
encounter with an old boyfriend she'd run into over the holidays, but
she refused to allow him to "pull out." "He finally just kind of rolled
over in disgust about the whole situation, and I said, 'You know,
that's just how it is.' "

Mechanical problems with condoms varied, from having difficulty putting them on (Dave, Donald), to having them slip off (Janice,
Hanan, Mary), to breaking (Susannah, Janice), to finding a hole
(Denise). By far, the most important difficulty was resistance to using
them. Among the straight and bisexual women and gay and bisexual
men, more than half had had experience with a man resisting condom use; one man (George) identified himself as resistant. Most
women found that assertiveness was sufficient to convince a man to
wear a condom, finding, "They'd rather wear it and have sex than
not wear it and not have sex at all." Denise's prospective partner
protested, " 'Are you crazy? I don't have any diseases.' And I'm like,
'Well, we don't know that.' " She found it "infuriating" that "they
come up with a lot of excuses to not do it where women always have
to seem to come up with excuses to do it."

Participants repeatedly stated that an argument over condom use
would be sufficient to spoil an encounter:

> Hanan: And then it would already have changed the whole mood of the
> whole thing because he'd start getting huffy and puffy, so it'd be like,

"Well if you want to stay here and spend the night and sleep here, feel free. But nothing's gonna happen, so if you're okay with that . . . "

DL: Have you ever had a guy say to you that he didn't want to use one?

Ginger: Oh yeah, actually, yes, I did—the guy was pretty forceful. He didn't want to use a condom and I kept stopping him. He didn't want to put on a condom, and I was just "Stop it!"

DL: And what happened?

Ginger: What happened was I just stopped it. And he's like "oh, okay, I'll put on a condom" and I'm like "No! Stop it!" I was getting really pissed off, and so that was it.

DL: So he stopped and he left, or what?

Ginger: No, he just stopped, and then we just hung out and talked for a while.

DL: 'Cause he didn't have one and you didn't have one?

Ginger: No, he had one, but I—it's too late, I just don't—'cause it's so frustrating to me to have to ask him someone to do it like seven times.

For Janice, her partner's resistance had become the defining issue of their relationship. She interpreted his resistance as a lack of concern:

Janice: I was under the pressure of him saying he didn't like condoms. I didn't want it to be an issue every time we had sex whether he was going to wear a condom or not. And it's still like that now.

DL: I was wondering if that had changed?

Janice: It hasn't. It hasn't changed from the first time we made love until now. We were at his cabin and were about to make love and he asked, I don't know, it just kinda felt like, you're clueless, you're dumb. I was afraid that when he said that I was just going to lose any desire. My arousal was just going to flatten out. And I tried not to think about it because I didn't want it to be a bigger issue than it was. But it's been affecting me.

Some women didn't like condoms for their own reasons, partly as a result of their partners' reactions. Sarita thought "it didn't feel as intimate," and her partner's complaints reinforced her distaste. Ann didn't like the effect of men's discomfort on their performance, "you get this friction, and then you've got to hear your boyfriend complaining, and they're jabbing all around like they don't know what they're doing because of the lack of sensation." She understood her partners' complaints as merely venting, because "it wasn't like if you complained loud enough I'd go, 'Okay, don't use it,' " but also asserted that "nobody uses them all the time." Susannah didn't like condoms because "it took forever for him to come, for one thing."

Because men are usually amenable to having sex but women usually decide when it will occur the first time, men realize that they need to be "prepared," even when they have not yet had intercourse. Rick had been advised by his father to keep one with him, so "I always had one with me just in case it would happen." Sarita's and Rita's partners carried condoms for their first episode of intercourse. The women had been involved sexually with their partners for some time before they would proceed. They described the first time they decided to have intercourse:

> Sarita: He had come up to visit, and I'd always held back, and I guess I was just ready. And we used a condom. . . . He had it.

> Rita: We never really discussed who'd bring the condom. I mean, in that department he was always prepared.

> DL: How did you know that?

> Rita: Because the first time we were fooling around and he took his condoms out. And I was like, "Oh, I don't think I'm really ready for that." He's a really responsible person when it comes to things like that. He's very conservative and he thinks things through sort of person.

> Hanan: The first time, he was very experienced, but you know I was a virgin, and he was very good about it, gentle about it, all those kinds of things, but yeah, he had the condom. He was always prepared about that, too. And this was—you know, AIDS was out already, it was 2 years ago.

Women were frustrated about men's resistance to condoms, but when men were "prepared," they interpreted it an indicator of responsibility and concern.

ADDING SPERMICIDE

As a result of the sex education they had received at Berkeley, Rita, Sonia, and Charlie began combining spermicide with condoms for contraception. For the rest, incorporating condoms was difficult enough; adding spermicide would have been even harder—"The condom is the easiest thing. It's one thing to use a condom and it's another to start using all the other different things like that." (Andrew).

Even though she and her girlfriend once discovered a hole in a condom, Denise expressed the difficulty of using spermicide thus:

> Even though I am up front and they need a condom, it's still, I mean I'm not saying that that's not hard for me to do, too, like if you're in the moment, I'm not saying that oh yeah, I'm so together that it's just really easy for me to grab it, I mean it takes extra, it really takes some extra pressure from yourself to say "Go get the condom," I'm not saying that it's easy for me to just be able to do that, but I know there is that extra little thing in me that says go get the condom, that's it. But now for me to be able to say go get the condom and the foam and everything else, it might be, that might be a little bit harder for me than just having the condom ready. . . . I have just gotten the hang of in the past couple of years incorporating the condom into being slightly erotic. But I mean, now this is something else that you have to deal with. I mean, it's hard . . . Why I would only use a condom? . . . Well I guess in my mind, using the condom, I would think well, maybe my rationale is I'm doing more than a lot of other people are doing, you know, I'm using a condom. I mean, that's what we were told to do, you know, that type of mentality.

Safer sex campaigns have been so focused on condoms that the word *protection* has become synonymous with condoms. When Lauren was in high school, "we didn't think of protection as that big of a thing, until we got to our senior year in high school. And then after that it was just like, 'you better use the condom, you better protect yourself.'" For many, condoms are sufficient protection (Lauren, Denise, Eric, Ginger, Shawn, Raphael, Andrew, Wheeler): "For now condoms is just what I'm using only." George, who wasn't concerned about STDs, considered condoms sufficient because they "trap the semen and there's just no way she's going to get pregnant." For Raphael, it was simply easier, "I have all these condoms and it's usually condoms that people pass out or give you, you know what I mean?" When I asked Hanan whether she'd used spermicide, she replied,

> No, I never, I've never been into foam. My um my gynecologist kept telling me about that too. I just always use condoms, lubricated and nonoxynol-9 kinda deal. Um, and right now I'm in a long-term, well for the most part, 9 months, monogamous relationship, so you know, I was going to but I, you know, I just kind of whatever, I'll get to it when I get to it, I'm not really that concerned about it at the moment.

Furthermore, for some women, the idea of using spermicide is as distasteful as condom use is for many men. The chemicals are perceived as harmful and unpleasant:

Ginger: . . . But then we always use protection.

DL: What does protection mean to you?

Ginger: A condom. It's enough protection.

DL: I ask everybody, everybody says condoms. Do you ever use foam? Or jelly?

Ginger: No. No. No.

DL: Just never occurred to you?

Ginger: Um . . . I want to use this . . . I, I just don't want all the substances on me, in me. It just—I'm weird, I, I don't like it. I think the condom is fine.

Susannah: No. We stay away from those, because I don't—that stuff takes off fingernail polish! And to me, I'm just like, "I don't know if I want that inside of me, if it does something to fingernail polish."

Marianna: The taste is really aversive to me and that is not gonna do it and I get numb.

As noted previously, some participants presented their behavior as calculated in terms of risk and benefits, whereas others didn't perceive possible threat in behavior that posed some objective risk because they considered themselves as consistently and carefully practicing safer sex.

GENDER, POWER, AND CONDOMS

Holland, Ramazanoglu, Scott, et al. (1991) argue that the assumption of many HIV-prevention campaigns that using condoms is a rational strategy that people can discuss and decide about prior to sexual intercourse ignores the social mores and constraints on individual behavior. They maintain that condom use involves a very complex process of negotiation. Heterosexual encounters, they argue (p. 128), are bounded by gendered power relations that define and limit negotiation between partners, whereas sexual negotiation and communication assume an equality of position across gender that remains largely unrealized. Within this framework, condoms may become a material symbol of the structural power imbalance that is reproduced among young couples. Asking women to carry and "use" condoms ignores this reality and their place in relationships between women and men (p. 129), where they may be the site of struggle over desire, reputation, and responsibility. A survey conducted by the American teen magazines *Sassy* and *Dirt*[1] in 1992 received nearly 18,000 responses. Validating Fine's (1988) thesis and the accounts of the participants in this study, it found that being seen as sexually experienced for a woman was still more stigmatized than being seen as sexually inexperienced. At the same time, both young men and women typically became sexually active at age 16 years, and both considered 16 the appropriate age for sexual debut.

Hanan noted that sometimes people beginning a relationship will peruse each other's personal belongings to see what kind of person they are. For that reason, she believed women, especially will view possession of condoms as proof that a man intends to have sex, which in turn reflects on the *woman's* character. Hanan had little patience for this attitude, for

> if you might have sex with them, you might as well be open about it. You're gonna be naked. If they're gonna be standing there naked with someone else, I don't think it's gonna be that serious of an issue to bring a condom. I figure if they're gonna be that open with somebody, then you might as well be open all the way with everything else.

Apparently, discussion about condoms almost never occurs before the condom is needed. Women might have condoms available in their purses (Vicky) or at home (Joanna, Janice, Denise, Marianna), but they usually left it to men to produce them. Among some participants, responsibility for producing the condom was dictated by the setting.

Sexual encounters are also potential sites of both pleasure and danger, yet American adolescents are rarely prepared for most of the dangers or any of the pleasures. Many women feel "embarrassment about every stage of condom use" (Holland, Ramazanoglu, Scott, et al., 1991). Fine (1988) noted that male sexual power can be threatened by a woman's insistence on her need for safety or satisfaction. Women are aware of the difficulty of balancing innocence with availability, reputation with desire. Being prepared for sex in advance—or even being seen to be prepared—still jeopardizes women's standing and safety. Furthermore, the spontaneity of passion can be undermined by the recognition of risk and responsibility, both in women's need to be swept away and therefore not accountable and men's desire to achieve orgasm once arousal occurs. Male sexuality is often presented to adolescent women as a train that cannot be derailed once engaged. Men therefore exert power when they are accepted as the initiators of sex, when they threaten the loss of the relationship if the young woman will not have sex, when they refuse to use a condom even when asked, and when they destroy a young woman's reputation by posting her sexual activity on a "list" and labelling her with epithets.

Strategies for Risk Reduction

Although participants thought of protection as synonymous with condoms, they actually employed multiple strategies to decrease risk. Strategies varied by sexual orientation, but they were essentially based on how much one trusted one's partner and might include attempting to choose a low-risk partner, reducing the length of exposure in an unsafe encounter, making risky behaviors safer, and getting a negative HIV antibody test result before engaging in unprotected sex.

STRATEGIES PARTICULAR TO GAYS AND BISEXUALS

No one had fully incorporated the use of barriers for oral sex, but gay and bisexual participants were far ahead of heterosexuals when it came to the use of latex. Janice realized that she might need to use condoms for fellatio if her relationship with a bisexual man became sexual, because, given his sexual and drug use history, she could "see that there's room for that in his understanding of what's necessary." Marianna had progressed the furthest in incorporating safer sex measures into her repertoire. Marianna enjoyed using latex gloves, had used a dental dam once, and believed she would be able to use them with her next partner. She had no problem using condoms for fellatio, explaining, "Oral sex with guys with latex isn't a big deal for me anymore." When Dave tried condoms for fellatio, he found the taste "nasty," although he realized that the condoms with spermicide he'd tried tasted worse than the strawberry and passion fruit unlubricated ones he had at home. Dave, Sebastian, and Donald preferred to have oral sex stopping short of ejaculation. Raphael had a positive attitude the time he tried a condom for fellatio. He told his partner, "You're gonna wear one too," and when his partner asked why, Raphael replied, "because it'll be fun." Jacob had also used gloves on occasion,

> Jacob: Not usually because there's never usually been digital penetration and stuff. But the times it's happened, I've used gloves.
>
> DL: So would you feel as easy about slipping a glove on somebody?
>
> Jacob: A lot of people are really kind of, "Well, wow." Actually, actually, my last partner was, he was just, he said he just couldn't believe like how, he was taken aback by the fact that I was so concerned. I didn't

give the impression I'm worried, or that I was worried about anything but it was just like I was very concerned and really cared about what was going to happen, what could happen or what was going on.

Dave, Leo, and Wheeler used condoms for anal sex. Dave, who had engaged in passive and active anal sex about four times each, used lubricant, wore two condoms, and required the same of his partners. Although he'd had unprotected sex once, Sebastian considered his sexual encounters "fairly tame," meaning oral but no anal sex. He'd never heard of anyone using condoms for oral sex, but because of the possibility of transmission, he'd been tested. He sat down with a partner and had a discussion about their respective histories. He felt that his partner's community activities conferred protection,

Sebastian: We sat down and talked like [we're doing now]. Um . . . I like to do that, I sit down and talk, I say, "Well, let's talk about how 'bout here's this issue." He said he'd been tested, and that he hadn't had sex since. And I told him I had been tested and also the same situation, he'd done a lot with it and usually practices safe sex, and—

DL: He'd done a lot with what?

Sebastian: Oh, with AIDS research and raising money and fund raising, and knew about it, and went to the conferences and stuff. So anyway we talked about that, and him going, and that type of stuff. I told him my situation and my last just briefly sexual experiences, and you know, and we talked about that. And then this is the first time before we ever had sex, and he said, well, at the end, you know, whatever, if you'd like to get together, you know, not like that, I don't remember exactly how he said it, but he's like, "Call me tomorrow, I'll be at work. And give me call. It's up to you, you, you know, it's your choice. And how you feel about it." And so I went home and thought about it and thought about it and thought about it, and the next day I called him and we got together.

They decided that unprotected sex was safe because both had been tested and neither had been sexually active since their tests; "I felt we were both monogamous, both safe, I trusted him, and he trusted me." For Raphael, trust came with a relationship. He had never used a condom for oral sex but abstained from oral and anal sex in a casual encounter and felt safer when he knew someone:

If we do something the first time we meet then I usually won't do anything. I won't give oral sex or anything. And then . . . in relationships this, um, where it's been a little longer or whatever and I feel, I don't know, I guess I probably shouldn't but I sort of trust the person more, and don't [use a condom].

Like Sebastian, Raphael felt that his partner's occupation and concern with Raphael's antibody status made him safer:

He also works in a medical research lab, where they do AIDS research, and so he seemed a bit more responsible, you know. Like working in that kind of environment, kind of made it—me feel more comfortable with it. But he seemed so, *he* was asking me had I been tested, this and that and this and that, and so I kind of figured that he was so he was being sort of like he's—it was almost like he was living in this fear, it was almost like he was.

Dave and Leo had tried condoms for fellatio but found the taste objectionable. None of the men regularly used condoms for oral sex, but several mentioned stopping before ejaculation. Leo explained his rationale:

I know all the studies are out there and I'm like the biggest AIDS paranoid, but if I feel comfortable with somebody and I feel like they've gotten their HIV results back and I can trust that they're not lying (if we didn't go together) I feel that's okay. I mean it's, I don't like sucking on latex or anything.

The strategy therefore includes calculating the risk of contracting an STD by engaging in fellatio without ejaculation and the benefit, in this case not having to suffer the taste of condoms, "I know it's not safe, but it's safe enough for me, I think" (Dave). Wheeler normally used condoms for anal sex but considered them unnecessary for oral sex. He balanced his risk similarly:

Well, just through my knowledge of HIV transmission and the epidemiology of the disease, and the risk factors associated with different activities. I've, my information that I'm working with is that infection, the risk of infection through anal intercourse is several degrees . . . it's much riskier to have unprotected anal sex than to have unprotected oral sex before ejaculation.

Donald, who was bisexual, didn't engage in fellatio to the point of ejaculation and had never considered a barrier with a female partner.

Donald: Yeah. There is oral sex. Um . . . But usually it's very it's not intense oral sex. It's casual, I don't know how you say that. Uh, it's it is there, it does happen, it's not with a condom. But it's not very frequent and it's not very um intense is the only way I can describe it. It's casual oral sex. I don't know what to say.

DL: Is there anything that would make you want to use a condom for it?

Donald: For oral sex? . . . Is there anything that would make me want to? . . . No, because generally if I don't feel comfortable enough . . . with the person not to, I won't, and it just doesn't, you know, it doesn't have to happen. And it's like never on the first, you know, encounter, it's always after I know the person.

DL: And what about with women?

Donald: Um . . . I think yeah, sometimes it happens the first time.

DL: So have you ever used dental dams?

Donald: No. Never. I don't know, it's, it's . . . It's not something that interests me. Saying all these things makes me feel really strange, because it's, it's, I've never actually put myself into this kind of context and heard myself say how stupid I've been, but . . . But yeah, I've never, never . . . .

DL: Well, I'm trying to figure out how—

Donald: No I mean it's fine, it's good that I'm saying it now because I'm going to be um rethinking a lot of things.

Denise said that she would avoid getting involved with a bisexual man. No one else described this strategy—some participants spoke of friends who even preferred bisexual men because they were perceived as more chic or that they would somehow be less likely to get hurt in such a relationship.

HIV ANTIBODY TESTING

I had anticipated that individuals might go for HIV tests before becoming sexually active with a new partner, but testing turned out to be much less important a strategy than I had assumed. Some of the men had considered testing, but Shawn was the only heterosexual man who'd been tested, as a result of the encounter described previously. Eric had heard of people around the dorm going down to get tested, but he didn't know anybody who had done so. Lauren, who had not been tested herself, described her partners' interest in her antibody status as rather indifferent, "They'd be just like 'you don't have HIV, do you?' And I'd be like, 'No.' " Charlie echoed Lauren:

I've never heard a guy or a girl say that's what they ask. I think the
farthest they ever have gone is they might ask if their partner's had
sex before, and maybe with who, or how many people. But that's it,
I've never heard anybody saying what's your history, you know, have
you ever had an STD? I've never heard that.

Among the participants, testing simply seldom occurred to the
heterosexual men, who might go years without a physical exam.
However, because women who have sex with men must deal with
the perpetual possibility of pregnancy, even young women know that
sexual pleasure can be hazardous; sexuality for them is already medi-
calized. When they become sexually active, they may consult physi-
cians for contraception or Pap smears; they must become accustomed
to thinking of their sexuality as both private and emotional and as
something for which they need to be tested and on which procedures
are performed. They know that precautions can fail for even the most
circumspect woman, and their experience with or awareness of pregnancy tests makes HIV testing a reasonable component of ways in
which risk is managed. Among the women, Sarita, Ann, Susannah,
Denise, and Marianna got tested as a result of their activities during
their first year at Berkeley. Denise referred to her sexual behavior that
year as "random," Marianna said she'd been "rampant." For the
women, testing would most often be used as reassurance before they
would go on the pill—it was very clearly a trust issue, a test that a
partner would have to pass. Both Hanan and Denise speculated that
if they were in a long-term relationship where they wanted to discontinue using condoms, they would need to first get tested with their
partners. However, when Ann got her test result, her reaction was
"We're free. We don't have to even try to be responsible because we're
free and we're together." Sarita was relieved to go on the pill and
discontinue condoms with her first partner, even though she realized
that taking it every day forced her to consider herself a sexually active
person. Susannah tested at her partner's insistence but was offended
by his request because she considered herself low risk. She was the
only one for whom this came up.

> Susannah: No, I did. I went and I got tested because when I was in college
> in San Diego I was going out with this guy and I don't know what
> he read or heard or whatever but then he knew how many people I
> had slept with and he was just like, "I'm not sleeping with you again
> without a condom." Because I was on the pill then. And we were
> having sex without, without condoms. And he, I think he had only

slept with one other person and he had used a condom and he was, "I don't want to have sex with you any more unless you go get tested." I'm like, I thought that it was ridiculous. From what I had heard about AIDS, HIV, whatever, I knew that I had never done intravenous drugs. And I didn't suspect that any of my partners had because most of them were pretty straight, clean, I mean, I don't want to say "clean," I mean those things, stereotypes of what people who do drugs are like, whatever. Naive, I guess. Maybe naive to the point where they wouldn't know how to, come across, how to get them, kind of thing, and so, and I didn't think that, I don't know, I rationalized it so that I thought, "This was, this was crazy but I'll do it." It's a good idea.

DL: When was this?

Susannah: I was a freshman in college. I thought, I would like to know. I would like to make sure that I don't have it. That was a long week. 'Cause you, it's weird what you start thinking about when you do something like that. And I was kind of resentful towards him because he didn't go with me to get the test taken. He didn't go with me to pick up the results. I mean, I'm sure he was busy doing whatever with school, classes, whatever, but still I was like, "You were the one who wanted me to go get this test." And the counselor, the interviewer, whoever, when I went in and he asked me questions about my sexual history and drug use and all that kind of stuff, he kinda chuckled, you know like, "Here's this girl. You slept with a dozen people, whatever, and you've never done drugs and you usually use a condom, and you've never had any STD," He's like, "You're really low risk." And I'm like, "Yeah." And he's like, "Just wanted to let you know that. How come your partner's not here with you today?" I was like, "He's busy." And he's like, "Well, you know, you should have him come down. Maybe he should get tested too." I'm like, "Well, I don't think that will be necessary but I'll let him know, him and his one partner he used a condom with but whatever." But it would have been nice if he would have come down for support anyway.

Andrew reacted similarly to Susannah's partner when a woman with whom he'd not been using a condom informed him that her last partner had not always used a condom, but in his case, "she was very cool about it. She went and got tested."

Testing is a safe sex strategy employed more frequently by gay men than straight people. Because AIDS initially appeared among gay men and was constructed as a gay disease (i.e., Gay-Related Immune

Disorder), the gay men in my group had thought most about the issue and comprised the highest proportion of those who had been tested and of those who had considered getting tested at 6-month intervals. Raphael, usually the active partner, had once engaged in passive anal sex without a condom, stopping before ejaculation. He told me that "I probably thought of using one, but knowing that I had just been tested and I hadn't been with anybody else, it didn't really bother me that much." Dave's current partner was testing for HIV every 6 months. Dave believed the man to be HIV negative, because "he said he would shoot himself if he were positive." Dave got tested when he started volunteering at the Free Clinic and the test became easily accessible. Both men tested for "reassurance." Dave encouraged friends to get tested but found "a lot of gay people are more willing to do it." Jacob tested, "just so I'd have peace of mind. I wondered, what if? Were there things like microscopic holes somewhere and I just didn't know? I figured it was better for me to know than to go on wondering." Leo used lubricant and spermicidal condoms for anal sex and tested between relationships. He and his partners discussed their antibody status before their first encounters.

Leo: Generally I'll ask them first, "Are you negative?" and they'll say, "Would you mind if you go get tested?" or "Would you go get tested for me?" and stuff like that. I don't phrase it, I don't know how I phrase it but I think I come off as a concerned . . . usually they offer.

DL: So would you get tested at the beginning of each new relationship?

Leo: If they ask. Usually I'll say the last time I was tested and I just told Willy I was tested in, right before we went to Baja, I guess in June, end of May. And I told him I'll go again. If you want me to go, I'll go. I told him exactly what I did.

DL: So you were tested at the end of May and you were with Doug until June?

Leo: Yeah.

DL: And before Doug, how long ago was the one before that?

Leo: I had been dating these two guys since last October-November until February they both . . . but we never did anything. It was just like mutual masturbation . . .

DL: Kissing and stuff?

Leo: Yeah. Well, not even that. Only with one of them. So yeah, so about a year, a year and a half, that's all I had been doing.

Leo understood that testing itself offered no guarantees, and that his responsibility extended to current and past partners:

DL: If it were a "committed" relationship, do you think you could trust each other enough to be monogamous enough so that you could do any kind of unprotected sexual behavior you wanted?

Leo: No. I wouldn't. No. Maybe after a year, after getting tested at least twice, probably I'd wait the other 6-month period three times. Maybe then—and I can't say that now. I don't know. I don't know him. Maybe 18 months from now I will feel like I know him a little better, hopefully. But even then, I don't know. I think with maybe a guy like him I would be able to trust him, but a guy like Doug who really felt it for, I know I wouldn't be able to trust him. Because he had been involved with some guy for 3 years and they were monogamous but he cheated. They told each other that "Oh, no. We haven't done anything. I've not been with anybody," and had unprotected sex. And that scared me so much.

DL: He had unprotected sex with his lover?

Leo: And he cheated on his lover and it's very, I know it's true that Doug cheated on this guy.

DL: So when they cheated, did they have totally safe sex, no body fluids?

Leo: No, I don't think so. I don't think so.

DL: Doesn't sound very monogamous.

Leo: Well, they believed that. I'm like, "How can you be such an idiot and do that knowing that you were cheating and you were gone for—" sometimes he would be gone for the whole summer and I don't know. I wanted . . . I almost blew up, not blew up, I don't have that kind of personality but I could not understand. People will tell you stupid things, right? How could anybody do that today? It just, it blew me away. And I thought this was an intelligent guy. Maybe love does something to you, I don't know. But I could not believe that. It was just awful and I thank god I had him tested before, before we did anything. And then I had him tested again. Well, I'm going to wait for him to get tested again. Because I told him, "Just because we're not going out doesn't mean that I don't want to know what happened." 'Cause we had anal sex—with a condom—but that's how I am. Fortunately I had the relationship, I continued having the relationship with him where we're still friends, we're close friends.

DL: So he'll let you know?

Leo: Yeah, and I'm supposed to let Willy know when he gets it done too 'cause Willy—he didn't ask but I told him I'd let him know. Because it was a concern of mine and I'd feel like if I'm involved with him that I should let him know either way, so. I think people are pretty good about that today—hopefully. The people I'm involved with I think generally are. Maybe I'm really naive and everybody's just hoodwinking me or something, I don't know. But . . . We'll see, we'll find out.

AMBIVALENCE ABOUT TESTING

Wheeler didn't discuss his testing history with new partners unless prompted. He acknowledged his fear of getting tested and said he planned to do it, explaining, "it's on my list for this semester. That's one of the things I am determined to do." He said,

It scares me. And I just have a lot of emotional issues around HIV. I'm very educated on it. I've taken courses on HIV and I've done work with the [Names] Quilt and HIV education and stuff like that and it still scares me to death. And I haven't been tested and I guess my, the rationale, the way that I rationalize that to myself is that, is that I haven't engaged in risky behavior and so I shouldn't have a problem. And I keep trying to kick myself in the pants to go and get tested. But it scares me.

Wheeler was not the only one to express some ambivalence. Those who hadn't been tested alternated, like Wheeler, between not feeling at risk and planning to test, saying that they "procrastinate" (Hanan), "lag" (Vicky), "didn't get around to it" (Joseph), hadn't "managed to set aside the time and create a schedule" (George), or were "too lazy" (Karen). Even among those who were nervous about their result, only a few had considered how they would respond to a positive test. Susannah found that "your idea of how mortal you really are really hits home I think." A couple of participants worried about how they would tell people about a positive result. Lauren thought the "hard thing" would be telling her parents. Sarita didn't have the "courage" to return for her results until 6 weeks after her test. She was concerned first for her boyfriend,

I didn't really think about *my* life. I didn't really think gosh if I'm positive how am I going to deal with it, I just thought of oh gosh that means I've passed it on to my boyfriend. That's the only thing I could think about. I—All I could think about was how would I tell somebody else that I've given them a fatal disease. It wasn't, it wasn't necessarily like . . . 'Cause I guess I thought you know well if I have it I have it, maybe I deserve it. Um because maybe I didn't take care of myself. I mean I don't think anyone deserves it but I didn't take care of myself but all I could think about was you know how could I give it to somebody I totally love. I just—I couldn't think about how I would tell this person at all.

Positive Attitudes Toward Safer Sex

Apart from a strategy of testing, several people enjoyed or thought they would enjoy incorporating safer sex techniques. Sonia enjoyed taking charge of the supplies, "I don't really wait around and rely on him to go and get the condoms or to get this. It's like I feel more comfortable knowing that they're there 'cause I did get them." She and her husband had been completely inexperienced when they met, so the safer sex demonstration in the UC health education class had improved their sex life. Previously, he'd go to the bathroom to put on a condom, but as a result of the class, she was putting on the condom, he was inserting spermicidal foam, and both were much more relaxed. Denise had learned to find condoms "slightly erotic." For Marianna, gloves had become "normal," they "made it easier to enter people and I wasn't hurting her anymore, my fingernails weren't hurting her anymore at all." Leo didn't feel that he was missing out because he was "really visual. I can just watch the man doing it, masturbating himself, and that does a lot for me." He liked

> the fact that, in a way it does force you to do a little bit more work in terms of getting, trying to get to know somebody a little bit better in terms of "What's your history?" I mean you start with family, then you go into relationships and you go to the sexual history and it's fun.

Jacob asked partners to help put his condom on and learned to put them on partners with his mouth, "trying to make it playful or exciting."

THE IMPACT OF HIV ON SEXUALITY

Participants adapted to life in the age of AIDS with acceptance or anxiety. Leo thought he could kiss someone who was HIV+, but if he knew that a potential partner were positive, he would view him differently. He welcomed the chance to get to know someone by going for walks on the beach and feeling like he didn't have to excuse himself for being "boring in bed" in the beginning of a relationship. One was forced to be more open about sex, "it's always, 'Okay. So what's the deal here? What do you do? What don't you do? What's your status? If you don't know, let's go get tested.' " He had determined that he would not "involve myself with anybody who I can't talk to—about that. They have no place in my life really."

Susannah felt encouraged to begin practicing safer sex. Lauren felt that Magic Johnson's positive serostatus had meant that "protection's becoming more of a bigger part of, if we're gonna do this we have to do this. People are taking it a lot more seriously than I think they used to." Andrew had accepted safer sex as part of coming of age in the 1990s.

Denise and Shawn reacted to the epidemic with anxiety. Denise felt safe in her relationship with another woman and reluctant to get involved with men for fear of the risk they posed. Shawn said that "AIDS scares the shit outta me, and I always just preach just wear condoms and make sure you're protected, and try to know your partner as well as you can." Donald's response was similar to Leo's but came from fear rather than acceptance. His anxiety had made him

> reluctant to talk to a lot of people that I would talk to just because I don't wanna deal with sex. Just in terms of what I'm willing to try and what I'm willing to do and how I have to be stand-offish about it for a long time before I let myself try something, I think is directly related to HIV.

Barriers to Safer Sex

IMPEDIMENTS TO SEXUAL COMMUNICATION

Scott and Griffin (1989) found the main reasons given for not using condoms, even when they were available, were "drunkenness, 'losing control and not caring,' and being worried about a partner's response to the idea," reasons reflecting this age and stage of development. However, communication difficulties are not unique to heterosexual relationships. Sabogal et al. (1991) listed the following reasons for having anal intercourse without a condom among the men in their sample of Latino gays and bisexuals aged 18 to 30 years in San Francisco, taken in the summer of 1990. In this sample of 100, men averaged 2.46 partners per month, 13.71 in the previous year:

	Percentage
I was really sexually turned on	51
No condoms were available	43
I was in love	40
My partner looked healthy	40
My partner was really good looking	34
I had been drinking or using drugs	31
My partner didn't want me to	29
We had the same antibody status	26
It was difficult to talk about condoms	17
Afraid that my sex partner would leave me	11
I was very sad or upset	11
I was under a lot of stress	11

The factors that militate against safer sex include those that relate to the evaluation of a potential partner as discussed earlier, lack of communication about sex between partners, judgment about the risk involved in a behavior or situation, lack of self control, the effects of alcohol, ambivalence about having sex, and the inability to consider alternatives to intercourse. Some of those barriers are illustrated in the discussion to follow.

Men were aware that their hormones could impair their judgment, particularly with an especially attractive woman.

> Andrew: Apparently they say that men, there's a chemical difference in your brain when you are aroused, and you just get stupid. And I actually find myself, I have it in me, but I do, to say, "Nope, no . . . wait."

Although Andrew had learned to control his drive, Shawn had not:

> I'm naked on top of her, I'm just going, okay, I better put my shorts on real quick because this is not going right, and I do not have a condom. But I was just looking at this most beautiful girl that I've ever been with and I was just going, oh my god. . . . That's the point where you lose your intelligence, that you lose your common sense, where you're at the point where you're so turned on and you're about to have an orgasm and you're with a girl, mixed with alcohol that you lose— that's where the common sense goes right out the door.

DIFFICULTY TALKING ABOUT SAFER SEX IN A NEW RELATIONSHIP

The controversy over school-based sex education discussed earlier illustrates the difficulty in discussing sex in the public sphere. Explicit materials are condemned by their communities, and there exists no language to talk about positive sexuality: words to describe body parts and sexual activities are either medical nouns; street slang; or nonspecific, vague euphemisms, all contributing to difficulty in both public and private discourse. In all kinds of relationships, early sexual encounters are often marked by signals and codes to protect the reputation of the woman or to save face in case one of the partners decides not to proceed. This muteness clarifies the explanation that sex "just happened," for talking about sex can be interpreted as consent before sex has been agreed to. Inchoate communication forces discussion of sexual history to be indirect, relative to the relationship rather than to risk. Construction of trust therefore may include not directly questioning a partner's past (Wight, 1992).

Many of these factors were cited by participants as making safer sex difficult to talk about. A relationship may have been established without prior discussion; raising the topic later implies a lack of trust. Sometimes a person hasn't decided whether the encounter will end sexually, more commonly among women than men. Even after the decision has been made, women may hesitate to acknowledge to themselves, much less to their partner, that they intend to have sex and want to talk about it.

> Sarita: I think it would only happen if two people were *really* good friends first. I mean *really* good friends, and then if the relationship became physical um . . . before it became too physical I think I would—just from everything I know now, and I guess I just know a lot and I'm really scared, but I would make sure I would talk to this person a lot. And I think it would take a long, I mean a *lot* longer time to actually have intercourse with somebody. Or not just intercourse but become sexually active in any way that could transmit a disease.

When sex is used to form a relationship rather than as an outgrowth of an existing relationship, it is more difficult to discuss its implications. Actually engaging in sex with a new partner can be less intimate than talking about it:

> Shawn: Okay. We're talking here about people that are a couple that's just like, just starting to get, just starting to have their first sexual encoun-

ter, really. And the last thing they're gonna want to do is become tricky with how they're gonna like—if they're debating about whether or not to have intercourse there's no way that the girl's gonna say okay well just here have, you know, make me, or give me some pleasure and I'll give you some pleasure and we'll, you know, you can give me a hand job, or you give me a hand job and I'll, you know, rub your clitoris or something like that you know and give you a orgasm or something like that. Because if that happens they're gonna jump—both jump right into sex, I mean it's . . . they're both trying to practice a little self-restraint and—especially the girl—and if you do that, there's the last thing they're gonna let you do is that, I mean, really.

Wyatt and Lyons-Rowe (1990) identified the egalitarian aspects of primary relationships that foster open communication about sexual desire and participating in the decision making about sex as important components of relationships that could enhance women's sexual responsiveness. Holland, Ramazanoglu, Scott, et al. (1991) suggest that the definition of men and women as sexual agents must be redefined to establish the kind of communication necessary to negotiate the boundaries of sexual relationships.

DIFFICULTY PLANNING FOR SEX

Ambivalence about sex makes it difficult to plan for. For Donald, who was bisexual, the rewards of a sexual encounter might not outweigh the implicit risk: "A lot of times I don't enjoy it, so I go away thinking 'I've just put my life at risk for something I don't enjoy.' So I tend to just try to avoid it if I can." He had planned in advance to have sex only once and had engaged in sex when a condom was not available, explaining, "One time we debated for a long long time and we were just too horny and couldn't stop." Ann found planning impossible even with her current partner, from whom she had contracted HPV (human papilloma virus, or genital warts).

Ann: I guess I could go to the store but it just hasn't happened that way. And so it was always sort of like when we wanted to use something like that we didn't have it. But then the only time we think about going to get it was when we already needed it and so it wasn't like we ever had the foresight to think, "It's 3 o'clock in the afternoon and I'm on my way home from school. Tonight I might go to the movies with Peter and we might go have sex so I think I'll go to the store."

DL: What prevents you from thinking that way?

Ann: I don't know, it just never really occurs to me until I'm already in the situation.

DL: What keeps you from organizing it in your mind to plan ahead? Or to realize ahead of time that sex is likely to happen?

Ann: It's just sort of I'm thinking about it when it's happening or when we're alone together or something like that. But it's not something that invades my consciousness on a daily basis. Usually I'm running around in the rat race trying to get everything done on time and, and do all this at school and make it to here before I have to go to there and worrying about homework and assignments and whatever so even when we do have plans it's sort of like if we have plans at 7:00 or something until 6:50 I'm sitting there frantically trying to get through another chapter of a book or something. I'm not sitting and combing my hair in the mirror and getting all prepared and perfect and whatever. I don't have time for that.

DL: Do you like sex?

Ann: Yeah.

DL: So do you think about it when you're sitting in a boring lecture or waiting in line at the photocopier?

Ann: No, usually in places like that I'm thinking about where I needed to be 10 minutes ago. Probably just about the only time that I'm really thinking about sex, like I said, is when I'm alone with my boyfriend. Not necessarily like we're alone in the bedroom or something. Sometimes when we're alone in some, some like random place I'll be all, you know. But usually just during everyday going through life during the day and stuff, there's a thousand other things I'm trying to remember. And I'm only coordinated enough to have a half accurate Do list and so I'm always trying to keep the other half of that Do list right in the front.

DL: So it's not something that's on your grocery list or your drug store list, go up this aisle?

Ann: No. I usually don't even have a grocery list, that's how bad it is. So probably if I was really organized and I had a grocery list and a drug store list or something then one time like, when we're actually about to have sex and didn't have anything then I'd be like, "Wait, stop. " And I could go write it down or something but I haven't quite gotten it that coordinated yet. . . . Someday we'll get it together. It'll be like, I don't know, all the cosmos will align and we'll go to the store and deal with it but by then we will have run out of condoms or something like that and then who knows what'll happen?

Ann had a particularly fatalist attitude, compounded by the fact that neither she nor her partner liked condoms and none of their friends used them. She had never been in a situation where she and a partner discussed what the sexual boundaries were, what behaviors were acceptable, or even what contraceptives they would use.

Sex may "just happen," especially with one considered a friend, although whether an individual will be prepared or willing to engage in unsafe sex in a spontaneous situation varies. Denise, though involved with Maritza, had had sex with a male friend,

> one of those friends who, we're really good friends and sometimes sex just happens. . . . But he knows my position, so he understands that if we are gonna engage in any type of sex it's gonna be safe and that's just how it is, because I just know too much now not to.

Donald's encounter with a female friend was not safe, however; "Well I kinda had a quick relationship, not a relationship, a night with the girl. It was a friend that was just that one night." With a male partner, "we met on Sproul steps just kinda sitting around . . . we didn't pretend to have more than a friendship even though at times it was sexual." Ann also enjoyed sex with friends and didn't plan because "in those situations, yeah, that was definitely a very spontaneous thing."

Apparently, the rules and circumstances surrounding sex with "friends" are different than those with "partners" and may involve even less advance planning and self-awareness. When Hanan had sex with a friend,

> it wasn't like I picked him up somewhere and then that same night I slept with him. It was like we had been friends for a long time and were were kind of doing the oh, maybe, maybe kind of thing, and then one night we did sleep together.

Because friends are viewed differently than lovers, risk is also perceived differently:

> Ann: No. Well, with my boyfriend now he's the first person I've been in a long relationship with. The other guys were people that I had to for a long time and still am, just friends with, and then it was just something that happened one night or a couple of times or something like that. And so we never really related to each other as a couple getting concerned about things like going down to get tested.

Among those who have difficulty planning for sex, spontaneity can be more important than risk. George had attitudes very similar to Ann's.

George: You can sit across from somebody and say stuff, but it's not, you know, I think the attraction human beings have to sex is the spontaneity of a situation and if you talk about it so much, there's a, Martin Luther King said this phrase, "paralysis by analysis." You know, if you over analyze the situation so much that it just takes the spontaneity out of it . . .

DL: So how do you balance planning and taking care of yourself with being spontaneous?

George: Well first of all, I'm not dumb enough to go out and sleep with somebody on the first night and have unprotected sex. No. That's first of all, how I would balance it. Second of all, if I sleep with somebody, before I sleep with somebody, I'm going to, or during, find out what's going on. First and second of all, I'm going to balance that out. I'm going to know and I'm going to get her to talk about what the experiences she had, just like what would happen. Okay, right at that moment I looked at her, she looked at me and we both kind of clicked and we said okay. Now, there was a small risk that for the initial 10 to 15 seconds or however long it was, that something could have happened. I think it's whether transmission of AIDS, whether STD, you know, there's a small risk and I think that's the question that you're asking. How to balance out, not touching each other at all, and wearing a full body suit condom, right, which takes away from spontaneity. Okay, so I think that for me . . . I always have condoms, first of all and they're always available for me to use. Even though I don't like them, they're always available, so I know I could always go back and use them and that's the bottom line so it's not preparing for an evening because, now you're getting into an issue of couples who completely prepare for a sexual encounter. You know, oh okay, well we're going to have dinner and then well when we get back if anything happens, let's prepare for it, and I think that it takes away from spontaneous in itself.

DL: But you keep a condom in case?

George: Yeah, I keep a condom in case, but I don't think you should go to an extreme where you say 9:00 we're going to have dinner, 10:30 we're gonna be in bed, 10:30 this is where we're going to be at.

UNPLANNED SEX

Because women usually determine when a sexual encounter will progress to genital intercourse, it can be difficult for men to be prepared.

> Shawn: This was like about our fifth or sixth time going out, and we went back to her place and she asked me to stay the night and so I said okay. I'd stayed the night before and not had sex with her. And I went back there and she came out with just, I went to her room and started kissing and all that kind of stuff, and she just started to like, she went, "Okay, I'll be right back," and she came back and she just had this unreal like just Victoria's Secret outfit on and I was going oh my god, and I was all . . . I'm like, oh okay. I want to have sex with this woman really badly. And so but unfortunately I did not have a condom with me 'cause I didn't even think it would be, that was stupid, in the beginning of the night, that this was gonna lead to anything like this. I just didn't think I had a prayer with that girl.

In Shawn's case, the woman had a condom in her apartment. But though she could change into lingerie and let him know that she had a condom, she couldn't verbally acknowledge her desire for sex, so she was unable to produce it. They ended up having intercourse without it. Donald's friend didn't have a condom nor had he been expecting the encounter.

> Donald: It wasn't intentional, I was walking her home from someone's house and I was planning to drop her off and it was just like, "Well, come in for a second," and . . .
>
> DL: And she didn't have any at her house?
>
> Donald: She didn't have any, which is really strange to me, 'cause I would have expected it, too, but she didn't. . . . Like I said I actually don't go looking, I would try, I would avoid it if I could. Somehow it comes up and I happen to be in positions where it seems like the right thing and, I don't know, it just happened.
>
> DL: So is there, . . . it's interesting 'cause it sounds like that usually you don't plan for it? You don't say, "Oh, we're gonna get together."
>
> Donald: . . . I don't think I've ever planned to have sex.

Perhaps because of women's inability to articulate their desire, men hope for sex but cannot plan for it.

For Denise, unplanned sex was part of a constellation of behaviors specific to being in her first year of university and not particularly gender related. However, for Ann, sex had to be unplanned, because it was "an id-dominated thing." Like Ann, Mary showed a certain passivity regarding sexual decision making. For her, sex always "just happened."

> Mary: Well, it was like, we don't—we hadn't even been going out for long like maybe a month, I remember it was like a week before my birthday. And um we were just like in his room, we were just messing around. And then just all of a sudden it just happened and I was like, I was kinda tripped out by it 'cause it just happened all so quickly, sort of a spontaneous thing. But then um after that, after that incident it just, you know, it just happened occasionally or whatever. And then when he came back, it would just happen. But then it seems like every time we, every time he came back, he would want to make it last, so he'd want to do it a lot.
>
> DL: Did you talk, you said the first time it happened spontaneously.
>
> Mary: Yeah.
>
> DL: Did you talk at all about contraception or safe sex?
>
> Mary: During. I said, "Stop, stop, I think you should go put a condom on" or whatever.
>
> DL: Was he inside of you already?
>
> Mary: Yeah. So it was kinda almost pointless.

In high school, in the case of Lauren and her friends, the risk became normalized with respect to pregnancy.

> Lauren: It just became a regular thing, almost, that we would take that risk—then when we were like 16, 17—15, 16, 17, we didn't really ask each other about whether we used protection or not. We just had sex, and it was like another month later, "You gotten your period yet?" And that was the kinda question, but it was kinda like that just seemed to be a burden that came with sex, 'cause even if we did use condoms, we still worried about being pregnant, so I guess sometimes we figured it just would just happen and we'd just take that chance, and hope we wouldn't be pregnant. And we usually, usually didn't think about it in the middle of sex.
>
> DL: So it didn't hold you up any?
>
> Lauren: Not too much.

Although Lauren became more aware when she reached university, both she and Andrew had both admitted to unsafe sex in "the heat of the moment" on multiple occasions.

ALTERNATIVES TO INTERCOURSE

When condoms are not available, it is difficult to consider alternative sexual expression. "That's great in theory, but it's more like you're sitting there and your goal is to have sex with her" and intercourse is the only act left (Shawn, Donald), or because "it just seems kind of awkward, like you're rejecting this person and want him back again" (Dave), because they lose commonsense when aroused (Shawn), or because the option simply wouldn't occur to them (Sarita, George, Lauren, Dave). Masturbation, tribadism,[2] and frottage, even oral sex, and other safer behaviors are not usually viewed as a viable end point. Negotiating alternatives takes a certain amount of trust and willingness to postpone gratification, which implies history. Shawn again, in the same conversation:

> That that would work more for people that have been going out for a while that completely trust each other. You know, I mean the girl's not gonna give up her control, her self-control. I mean if this is like a relationship that's just started, I mean this is a typical relationship, that maybe guy and girl meet, you know, after 2 or 3 weeks or maybe a month or something, or 2 months, you know . . . Well, 2 months is a little different. But after a month or something like that, you know, they finally, you know, like start to get down and get to the point of where they're about to have sex, and they're not fully sure about their partner—I mean they're not completely trusting their partner at this moment they just met like 2 weeks ago, you know, the girl's not gonna say, "Okay, do everything you want to me except have sex with me." I mean she's gonna say, you know, sh—probably it's gonna be difficult just to have, like to . . . It's gonna be very difficult just to get to that point.

Marianna was the most conscious about the need for safer sex in multiple domains, yet even she found it difficult, saying, "I still have a hard time figuring out how to negotiate, like insisting on people being safe when they go down. I don't know how to do that yet." She could insist on condoms with intercourse with a casual male partner but had not been able to extend it as far as she wanted with her female partner, beyond getting over negotiating in the moment, his judgment of me is not gonna affect my self-image at all, whereas her judgments of me affect my self-image in a really out-of-proportion way. So telling her something that I think she might think bad of me for is really much more terrifying than someone I don't know.

DENIAL AS A DEFENSE

To reconcile their dissonant feelings, George and Ann questioned the validity of the data.

You can get statistics from one set of people and get them from another and they seem to contradict and some say, oh many heterosexuals are dying of this, and I'm going, "Okay, how many is many? And what's your sample?"

Even though George had told me that he was influenced by his brother's experiences, his brother and friend had contracted STDs, yet George refused to be swayed:

All that we have are these statistics and I think statistics are very very impersonal. You don't know where they came from, you don't know who did the study, you don't know the bias rates, you don't know the environment, all you have is a number like, like at Berkeley, on the average one out of four by the time they graduate, get their bachelor's degree have contracted an STD, I find that on the average one in four—to me that seems really really high, okay—one in four out of what, who are you studying, are you studying all ethnic groups, are you studying male, female, what are you studying on the average?

They seemed aware that only by feeling risk personally would they be able to attend to the messages, even when they themselves had contracted STDs other than HIV:

Ann: Statistics might tell you that you are at risk or whatever but statistics don't scare you. It's the personal things that scare you into changing. And so like some of the, I think that having speakers just talking about what it's like instead of seeing these bar charts and graphs about like number of HIV positive and number of people with AIDS and those who have died, you know, all those line graphs tell you about it but it's not personal enough to get, to really drive the message home. So you might know all of this scientific knowledge or whatever but you don't have that emotional component that's telling you, seeping into your conscience.

Ann acknowledged that it would be almost impossible, however, to make that risk personal for her. She had the most fatalistic attitude of all the participants, coupled with clear insight that made her attitudes that much more exasperating, and worth quoting at length:

> Ann: I think there's a big difference between something can be very effective, you know, scaring you and making you aware of what's at risk, whatever, but it still could be very ineffective and actually when it comes down to it, in that situation when it's just you and that other person getting you to change your behavior, and so I think that part of the AIDS thing is people think it's big giant thing beyond their control, kind of like a natural disaster or something. It's like if you live in California you've got to expect there's gonna be an earthquake so when your house falls down because of an earthquake, you can't complain.
>
> DL: Does that mean that you shouldn't earthquake-proof your house, or get earthquake insurance?
>
> Ann: It, yeah, but you could go around and ask how many people have earthquake insurance and it's probably not as many as it should be. Everybody's got home insurance but all these policies that don't cover earthquakes. And that earthquake insurance costs more and so you don't do it. It's like you'll do the minimum required but you won't do that extra whatever. I have a scooter that's an old classic and trying to get insurance for it, you just want the cheapest policy. You don't care what it covers and what it doesn't cover. You just want the least expensive policy. And so, it's kind of silly, 'cause, well, if you're gonna get your insurance or whatever you should get what's actually gonna be worthwhile or useful and you shouldn't be worrying about the other costs because in the end like if you're really that worried it'll pay off.
>
> DL: And how would that relate to sex, do you think? To continue your analogy.
>
> Ann: That people don't perceive that that extra caution is gonna pay off because it's sort of like this force that's gonna happen to them or not happen to 'em. It seems so random that how could you control it anyways? And so people don't perceive that, the efficacy of their behavior is nil. It's like, "Well, I could change my behavior but it's not gonna change anything." People think they're immune. "It's not gonna happen to me." We all think that. We all want to believe that.
>
> DL: Do you think it would make a difference if you knew somebody who was positive?

Ann: It might well. Definitely, that might make a difference. But then again, I think it would make a difference in that I'd still be yet more aware but I don't know, when it comes down to the behavioral level, how much that would do because I could very easily see knowing somebody who's positive and just saying like, "They only had sex with one person once ever and they got it and so how did it happen to them?" You can use it as, both ways. You can look at it and see what a horrible disease it is and then try to, try to avoid getting it yourself or you could look at it and go, "That person did everything right and they still got it."

DL: So there'd be always some way to make a person not like you.

Ann: Yeah, and there's always gonna be, you know, you look at the, the kids who are positive and then you break it down into the "innocent" people who did everything they were supposed to and nothing wrong and still got it and other people who were like didn't protect themselves ever and got it and so like you expect them to get it because they did everything wrong. And then there's the people that, that seem not to get it. When you can't make sense what it is, it's the "just world" phenomenon. When the people who get it and they don't deserve to get it and you can't explain that and so then you just, because people want to believe that, you know, people only get what they deserve to get.

DL: What kinds of people who get it sexually deserve to get it or don't deserve to get it?

Ann: Well, nobody does deserve to get it. But, I guess, in, in my image, it's the people who, I guess it doesn't really make sense, but then again, none of our little schemes actually make sense when you try to explain 'em. I mean, you just are taking home lots of different people every night that you just barely know, things like that. And I don't know how that's really different from just sleeping with somebody you already do know, but it seems different. There's that line there. And so, people who take home a lot, a lot of people, multiple partners, because that, I guess, it seems like for, it's just one of those exponential things where if you're taking home lots of people and they're also the type of people who also take home lots of people then pretty soon you've slept with all the West Coast.

When we consider young people fatalistic or in denial, it may be appropriate to question the model we employ in defining risk. Clearly, some people know what objective behaviors put (other) people at risk, but don't necessarily apply it to their own situation. The construction of risk entails more than a public health understanding of potential morbidity associated with risk behavior.

ALCOHOL AS A BARRIER TO SAFER SEX

Last, alcohol is one of the greatest barriers to safer sex. Men may enjoy its disinhibiting effects (e.g., George: "I think that alcohol adds to sexual activity enormously") but for women, it is alcohol rather than hormones that clouds their judgment and affects their ability to assert themselves in a sexual situation. Half the women talked about sexual situations in which they or their friends had been involved that would not have occurred had they been sober. Ann engaged in a menage à trois with two friends, which she wouldn't have had she not been "really drunk," and on another occasion, drank to overcome the awkwardness of a relationship in transition from coworker to sexual partner. Similarly, Vicky used it for the permission it gave her to be with a man other than her primary partner:

> We went out maybe two times after that but we went out like more than friends those two other times and on this third occasion—see, I haven't gone out with him that long—I mean it's not like I was totally cheating behind my boyfriend's back, but still, it's not, moral anyhow, so I went out on that one day and well, see, this is really bad—I got like, not drunk, but pretty buzzed and tipsy that night and we went back to his place and we were just playing music and just laughing, talking and he opened up another bottle of champagne. It's getting pretty bad here but the thing was I think at this point, I don't know, I think because I was under the influence, that I wouldn't have mind if we, you know, did have sex and the whole time was rushing through my mind but the whole time I was thinking, like, well, if this does happen then if he does ever cheat on me, then I would have had the first—you know, it's really bad and that's not the kind of relationship I want but that's the kind of relationship I was in, where it's like a game to make sure you don't get hurt first.

Drinking to the point of not remembering what one had done was not uncommon. Marianna said she'd "had sex a couple of times because I was too drunk to deal with not having sex." Lauren contracted HPV from such an encounter:

> I thought I got 'em from this guy that I slept with on my birthday, 'cause I got so drunk, I didn't even know I was with him. And all of a sudden I kinda came out of it, and here I am with this guy, and I was just like "aagh!" 'Cause I didn't even realize—'cause at a dance place,

and it was my 18th birthday, and it was like, I first got to the dance place and the bartenders were like, "Go ahead, but don't hold onto the drink, 'cause I'll have to kick you out." So they're like "drink it fast." Boom. It was Long Island Iced Teas and all that stuff. And I'm a lightweight, two beers, I'm buzzed, off the wall, you know. And I just drank three or four of 'em, dancing, next thing I knew I'm up by the balcony getting it on with this guy. And I was just like "ugh." Then I was trippin' after that, 'cause I couldn't believe that where I was, I have never been so drunk to where—'cause I don't drink that much, to where I just didn't, it was straight blackout. I didn't know I was there and then when I came back and all of a sudden I'm with this guy, it was just aagh!!

Denise narrowly escaped rape when she got drunk at a fraternity party:

I went to a house, and he said "Well, come here I want show you the game room." I was drunk, fine, let's all go to the game room. And we went into this room, it was completely dark, and he shut the door. And it's a door that doesn't open from inside. So once you're in you're in. And so I started to get a little bit more sober 'cause I realized where I was at, and um he started kinda like pressing me up against the wall type of thing, he was like, "come on," you know, "this is the *game* room," and really I was drunk to the point where I didn't know what he was saying, but I knew what he wanted. And you know, he started taking off my clothes, and I was like, "No, I need to go." And so I went for the door, I couldn't open the door 'cause they have it rigged. The fraternity knows that this is the room to take women. And the only way you can get out is if you yell to the guys down the hall. So I was yelling for someone to let me out of the room. And um he's like, "come on," you know, and I was drunk, and I was getting dizzy, and so I mean out of the blue Maritza and another friend of mine in the sorority who's, I was actually close to, her and some other guy that they found at the party came and he kicked down the door. 'Cause they somehow found me.

Date Rape and Coercive Sex

The line is slim between drinking too much and being taken advantage of and being date raped. The issue of date rape and coercive sex is important in the discourse of sexual negotiation because it reflects the impact of gender roles, sexual communication, and power in sexual situations. In the United States, there was debate at the time of this study in which some members were attempting to define date rape as little more than a communication issue. The difficulty with

defining the issue in terms of communication and miscommunication is that when date rape occurs, the woman is often held responsible for not avoiding the situation or for engaging in behaviors that
the man would consider provocative, effectively relieving him of responsibility for his actions, for as Sarita said, "by going upstairs with
someone you pretty much consent." There is little latitude for con-
senting to some behaviors but not others.

Marianna, Theresa, Sebastian, Leo, and Lauren had had experience with date rape or coercive sex; Hanan, Janice, Rick, and Charlie
had seen friends through it. I didn't interview any men who admitted
to date rape, but George gave me his opinions on sexual miscommunication.

> George: But sometimes if you talk about it, right, it's the communication
> factor between sex is so difficult because there have been times where
> someone will say, you, know, I don't think this is what we should be
> doing. And I've been in a situation where the woman says, "Well, I
> don't I don't think that we should be doing this," questions it, then
> continues, continues physically, continues with the kissing, contin-
> ues with the fondling and continues, but expresses, now this is some-
> thing that I'm really interested in is the date rape occurrence. Now
> is that rape? If a women says no, okay, but continues, it's really in-
> teresting, in fact, we had this question in class, where we did a values
> continual [sic] and this question was read. The situation where a man
> and women are engaged in sexual intercourse and the women says
> no, however, she continues, has the man raped her? And I was the
> only one on the other side of the room because I think that the man
> didn't rape her. I think there's something more there. That the
> woman is not communicating herself effectively, she might say no,
> no verbally, but she's not saying no physically, she's continuing do-
> ing these things, I think rape occurs if she says "no, I don't think we
> should be doing this," and says "No, we need to stop," I think "Please
> stop what you're doing, please stop touching me, we need to talk."
> Okay, if she continues to do this, but I've been in situations many
> times, I will tell you, many times, where I've been engaged in sexual
> activity and the woman says, "Well, I don't think we should be doing
> this," however continues and I continue.
>
> DL: What do you think she means when she says "I don't think we should
> continue," if she—what is she trying to express when she says that?
>
> George: In all honesty, I think she's trying to express that society would
> not accept her doing that but she physically as an individual needs

to and she knows that in society's eyes, wow, this might be bad because I'm having sex with some guy, whether it was unprotected, whether it was you know, on the first night or what, this societal views come in but as an individual, as an individual, she likes it, she thinks it's great, she feels comfortable physically, right, but all of a sudden it comes out "I don't think we should be doing this" because society said it was wrong, then I question—what goes through my head is why do you continue to touch me then, why do you continue doing this? If we stop and all of a sudden you continue fondling me, why are you doing that, you know.

DL: Have you had anybody say, you know, I want to just fool around. I don't want to go all the way?

George: Yeah.

DL: So let's just fool around for a while, but then I want to stop.

George: Beforehand, or during or when? Whenever?—yeah. I mean I respect that, I'm not, you know, I'm not somebody whose out to just screw somebody.

DL: No, you've already made that clear.

George: Yeah, but I respect that, but I think it's too late. Now this is the question that was asked: if they're already engaged in sexual intercourse, by then it's too late.

George's view of communication and a woman's right to say no contrasted with Lauren's experience.

Lauren: Yeah. I was raped once. I was date raped. Yeah. I was going out with this guy for like a month. And um, we got in a fight, we were at my friend's house, and there was 10 of us there and we'd all been drinking, so I wasn't, I hadn't drunk 'cause I wasn't drinking then. And um we got in this big argument. We went in the bathroom. Their bathroom was like really big bathroom, it was this big house. And we were talking it out, arguing it out and everything. And then we just started making up, started kissing and everything. And he—we hadn't had sex yet. And he knew I didn't want to have sex. Because I'd just gotten out of a relationship and I wanted to wait, you know, and this whole bit. And then um we were just like kissing on each other and doing all that and he kinda just kept going. And I didn't really trip at first and then, then he was just like bam. Was inside me. I was like, "Uh-uh. Get out." I was like, "Stop stop stop."

DL: So you were on the bathroom floor?

Lauren: Yeah. And we were just like kissing and hugging and touching and stuff, and then he just, and then he just got between my legs, boom, went in, and I told him, "Stop it, I'm not ready for this, I don't want to do this." And he didn't stop. Then he pinned my arms down and kept going. And then he got up and he was like, "You're all dry." And he took some water and put water on me and came back down and did it again. And I was just like, yelling at him to stop. Then finally my friends banged on the door, they're like "Are you okay?" I was like, "No!" And so I got out and I was all upset, and he was like, "What did I do?" I said, "I told you to stop" and everything. He was like, "I did stop."

DL: How did he think he'd stopped?

Lauren: I know, I don't know. 'Cause I told him to stop stop stop stop and finally, STOP *STOP* **STOP!** And he finally stopped.

DL: Is that what brought your friends, 'cause you were yelling? They didn't hear you before that?

Lauren: No. They kind, they heard something but they didn't know what it was. And I was talking to my friend, 'cause one of my friends was there, so then we were just talking about it, she said, "It's like I knew something was going on but I didn't know what to do, so I didn't do anything." She says, "And I'm always gonna regret that 'cause I know what he did to you." And I was like "Well." And they were like "We're sorry we didn't come in sooner." And it's like, well it's over, it's done now. And I was just, I couldn't drive, I couldn't, I was just upset. And we just left, and I told my friends what happened and everything, and he called me back later that night. And he was totally crying, and he was like, "How could you think I did that to you?" I was like, "You *did* it." I was like, "And don't ever call me again." And then, the next guy I went out with, he would start to get together with me and I just started crying. Then I had another boyfriend after that, and I, any time he'd come even close to touching me I started crying. And he was like "What happened to you?" And I told him, he was like, "I'm gonna kill him." Then he told me he killed him. And then the guy who raped me, he called me up, he says, "I still have a place for you in my heart." And I was like, "You're supposed to be dead." But I didn't say that. I said, "Don't you *ever* call me again."

DL: What do you think he thought happened? If he were to tell the story, what do you think he would have said?

Lauren: I think he probably would have said "I don't understand what went wrong, 'cause we were just, I just wanted to make love to her and so that's what we were doing and then all of a sudden she just, she just started crying on me," or something. That's probably what he would think. 'Cause it seemed like he was just completely out of the whole picture. Like I looked at him it seemed like he just didn't hear me, or just didn't . . .

DL: Did you think of trying doing something physical?

Lauren: Yeah. I was, I was trying to get away, and he had my arms down. And then he got up, when he got up, I was just so shocked that I didn't get up right away. I was just stuck. It sounds like what is he doing now? And then he came back down and I was just like unngh. 'Cause as soon as he got down—'cause he was a lot bigger than me, too. So I was just like, ugh. So I was trippin' after that.

Lauren said she was "really promiscuous" for a while after that. Promiscuity after date rape was a recurrent theme; for example, Charlie's friend began "having one night stands, sometimes she doesn't really know them, she just met them once. And at first I was really disappointed. But then I was thinking about what happened to her during the past year." Date rape and sexual abuse can provoke either abstinent or so-called promiscuous behavior; it is the latter that presents a risk for STD transmission where women (or men) don't protect themselves as a consequence of coercive sex.

SCRIPTED REFUSAL, DOUBLE BINDS, AND THE SEXUAL DOUBLE STANDARD

Wight's (1992) analysis of the reasons for lack of verbal negotiation before intercourse corroborates that of Muehlenhard and McCoy (1991), that in spite of greater sexual freedom today, women still feel obliged to tell a new partner that they don't want to have sex when they do. Men therefore learn to not accept a refusal as definitive. These investigators found that a significant proportion of incidents among women who had initially refused sex when they wanted it (which they called *scripted refusal*) ended in sexual intercourse. In about half of those cases, the woman indicated that she changed her mind, but in the other half, she had never indicated her willingness to have sex. Among the women labelled as engaging in scripted refusal who proceeded with intercourse, most felt badly about it, yet they thought their partners reacted more positively than they would have if the women had refused. The only factor that predicted scripted refusal was a woman's perception of her partner's acceptance of the double standard. They found that men subscribed to the double standard more than women, and women believed that men accepted the double standard even more than they did (p. 458). Shotland and Hunter (1995) found that after some weeks of a dating relationship, many women offered only "token resistance" at the point at which they were deciding to engage in more intimate sexual activity. George made it clear that when women continue to say "no" when they mean "yes" and then accede to intercourse, men become unable to distinguish between scripted refusal, token resistance, and rape. Moreover, "where men see sexual negotiation as a process of attrition, as wearing a woman down until she says yes, there are problems in producing a condom at the right moment" (Holland, Ramazanoglu, Scott, et al., 1991). A double bind is thus created for both sexes when women suffer negative sanctions for their open acknowledgment of desire.[3]

Date Rape, Coercion, and the Negotiation of Consent

The issue of date rape is crucial to the understanding of the construction of sexuality and sexual negotiation on campus, both in and of itself and in its relation to risk for STD. With regard to the current study, the issue is an exemplar of the difficulty of gendered power relations and failed sexual communication. Although it does not represent a major part of this research, it is part of the issue and worthy of further study in its own right. I will not review all the analyses of date rape here but will refer briefly to the controversy between those such as professor of social work Neil Gilbert and postfeminist media personality Camille Paglia,[4] who at the time were publicly commenting that date rape scarcely exists, and various feminist scholars, who situate date rape in the general field of violence against women.

The context for date rape on campus is often similar to that of consensual sexual relations; fraternity parties and presence of alcohol are thematic in both, for example. During the time of this research, there was active debate at Berkeley on the prevalence and definition of the problem, precisely because the boundaries of resistance and consent were sometimes blurred, as Lauren and Denise described.

Date rape is sometimes distinguished in the literature as different from acquaintance rape. The latter may include a broad range of coercive partners and situations. I am primarily referring here to coercive approaches that occur in social situations in which sexual negotiation might occur, such as dates or parties, but not those that may be perpetrated by someone outside of these situations—for example, a study partner or the mail carrier. In November 1991, Diana Russell, law professor and author of many works on violence against women,[5] gave the Seabury Lecture at UC Berkeley's School of Social Welfare. Her talk, titled "The Epidemic of Sexual Assault Against Women," largely addressed an article by Neil Gilbert, UC Berkeley professor of Social Welfare, in the campus' Spring 1991 *Public Interest.* In this article, he maintained that rape statistics are inflated out of proportion and that what was being identified as a date or acquaintance rape epidemic was little more than miscommunication between sexes. Gilbert (1997) believed that antirape activists are engaged in "an effort to reduce the awesome complexity of intimate discourse between the sexes to the banality of *no means no*" (p. 11). Gilbert was present at the lecture and offered a lengthy rebuttal to Russell's arguments.

Gilbert was criticized by Russell for having done no primary research, instead, using rape statistics gathered by the Bureau of Justice Statistics Department, which estimates annual incidence of rape and attempted rape at .1%, or a lifetime prevalence of 7% to 8%. Moreover, he confused incidence with lifetime prevalence, which Russell and many others cite at about 25%. Russell pointed out that her questions screened for rape as defined legally, whereas Gilbert's had been based on Bureau of Justice phone survey questions that were sufficiently vague to not pick up women who had been raped according to its own definition. These questions did not specifically mention rape or sex, and the Bureau itself later determined that the questions should be revised. Koss (1992) concurred with Russell's prevalence figures, noting that critics of surveys on date rape, such as Gilbert, err in their assumption that a broad definition of rape undergirds the empirical data base. Date rape critics further assert that the large discrepancy between the estimated rape rate for college students by Koss (1992), Russell, and others, and estimates by the 1991 National Crime Survey (NACS) (Bachman, 1994) casts doubt on the validity of the former. This assertion fails to take note of the criticism that the NACS approach to rape measurements has received in the literature. This criticism has focused on the wording of the NACS rape-screening item. Disbelievers in date rape exclude women who do not think they have been raped, even when their cases fit the legal definition of rape. Although critics assert that nothing should be called date rape unless so designated by the victim, Koss (1992) maintains that this assertion reveals unfamiliarity with victimization survey methodology.

Copenhaver and Grauerholz (1991) and Koralewski and Conger (1992) noted that college women are at high risk of rape or attempted rape, confirming Koss's (1992) and others' 25% lifetime prevalence rate. Among college women who had been subject to this type of assault, half the perpetrators were dates, 35% acquaintances, 10% friends, but the majority of women had been further subjected to some form of force, the least offensive of which was described as "unwanted sex play excluding intercourse." Ogletree (1993) surveyed midwestern college women and found that nearly 50% had been exposed to some form of coercion, mostly in the form of giving in to sex because of a partner's unrelenting pressure and arguments. Sorority women are at particularly high risk because of their association with fraternity members, although Copenhaver and Grauerholz (1991) were careful to note that if the sorority women spent as much time with nonfraternity men, they might be equally at risk; nevertheless, they concluded that the fraternity environment supports sexual coercion.

Alcohol plays a large role, according to these authors, because its disinhibiting effects serve as a catalyst. Abbey (1991) found that drinking and date rape were related because men expected intercourse to occur in a date involving drinking and felt justified to use force when women resisted, because it affected women's ability to send and receive cues and to resist sexual assault, and both men and women believed that women were more responsible than men for whatever happened in such situations. Before the alleged date rape, 79% of women and 71% of men had been drinking or taking drugs directly. Among those with whom the aggressor was a fraternity member or the act had occurred at a fraternity function, 96% of respondents and offenders had been drinking or taking drugs before at least one of the incidents. The more involved in sorority life a woman was, the more likely she was to have experienced coercion. In Abbey's study, 17% of the women reported incidents that legally qualified as rape. Between .8% (Muehlenhard & Falcon, 1990) and 2% (Copenhaver & Grauerholz, 1991) reported to the police, 5% to a rape crisis center, 7% to medical personnel, 10% to parents, 7% to relatives and none to school officials. Yet when those whose experiences met the legal definition of rape were asked "Have you ever been raped?" only 36% considered that they had, although another 32% were unsure, rebutting Gilbert's argument concerning legal definitions of prevalence.

The University's police department had only two rapes reported on the Berkeley campus and in university housing between January and October 1991, three in 1990, and one in 1989, the period before this study began. Although the number of reported rapes appears low, the number of women with unreported rapes presenting to various clinics served by the University Health Service (UHS) leads the

UHS to consider date rape by itself and combined with alcohol use to be problematic on the Berkeley campus (P. Flynn, personal communication, February 24, 1994),[6] as it is on university campuses throughout the United States (Sanday, 1990).

GENDER DIFFERENCES IN PERCEPTION
OF SEXUAL CUES AND COERCION

Many of the widely used paper-and-pencil tests among college students find that men consistently view women's behavior as more sexual than women do, that men's perceptions of how much a woman wants sex are consistently higher than women's, that men feel that coercive sex is more justified than women do, and that men regard "forced sexual encounter" as less serious than women do (Foley, Evancic, Karnik, King, & Parks, 1995), suggesting notable gender differences in interpreting male-female interaction. Muehlenhard (1988) found that men interpret who initiates a date, where the couple goes, and who pays the dating expenses as cues indicative of how much a woman wants sex. Abbey (1982) found that men viewed both men and women in more sexualized terms than did women and judged women as more promiscuous than women did. She suggested that because men view the world more sexually than do women, they are likely to interpret women's intended friendliness as seductiveness.

Where women and men interpret dating behaviors differently, there may be serious repercussions. If a man interprets a woman's initiative as a sign that she wants sex, he may feel led on if he finds that she doesn't. Sawyer, Desmond, and Lucke (1993) found that college men were more likely than women to perceive their partners as dishonest and likely to give misleading messages regarding sexual intent. Unfortunately, according to Muehlenhard (1988) and others whose work she reviews, many males regard being led on as justification for having sex with the woman against her will—in other words, as justification for rape. Undergraduates were more likely to think a woman wanted sex, and rape more justifiable, when she initiated the date. Among Muehlenhard's students, men's ratings of how much a woman wanted sex, given a particular scenario, were always higher than women's. In their studies among college students, Bell, Kuriloff, and Lottes (1994); Sheldon-Keller, Lloyd-McGarvey, West, and Canterbury (1994); Holcomb, Sarvela, Sondag, and Holcomb (1993); and Lenihan, Rawlins, Eberly, and Buckley

(1992) found that men also thought that rape was more justifiable than did women.

Students in Muehlenhard's (1988) study who were labelled "traditional" or "nontraditional" rated how much a woman wanted sex almost equally when the man asked the woman out but diverged as the woman took a more active role; when the woman asked the man out, traditional persons rated the woman as more willing to have sex than did nontraditional persons. Traditional men rated rape as significantly more justifiable than did nontraditional persons. Muehlenhard (1988, p. 33) hypothesized that traditional men may be more likely than nontraditional men to feel led on and thus to feel that rape is justifiable. Perhaps both would be equally likely to feel led on, but traditional men are more likely to believe that being led on justifies rape. Hence, this study explored whether subscription to traditional gender roles affected the ability to negotiate sexually.

Koralewski and Conger (1992) assessed social skills among non-coercive, moderately coercive, and coercive college men, evaluating consensual and coercive sexual experience, social skills, assertiveness, and attitudes to coercion. They found no difference among groups on self-report or performance measures of social competence; this is perhaps not surprising, because the men had to be dating to qualify for the study and, therefore, would be expected to demonstrate a modicum of social skill. However, like Muehlenhard and Falcon (1990), they found differences among groups for measures relating to sexual callousness and acceptance of interpersonal violence against women, further supporting previous research in the field. Muehlenhard and Falcon found that men with high sexual dominance scores were more likely to have managed sexual intercourse through coercive means, including arguing, lying, getting a woman drunk, or raping her. They found that men with traditional gender role values were more likely to have engaged in verbal coercion ending in intercourse. However, Porter, Critelli, and Tang (1992) found only "sex guilt" to be a measure of sexual aggression, predicting the amount of force used. More research is needed to evaluate these and related hypotheses about differences between gender role identification and attitudes toward rape.

Canterbury, Grossman, and Lloyd (1993) found a date rape rate of 3% among incoming first-year female students and 2% among incoming males, with a higher lifetime prevalence among those who drank 2 to 4 times per week. In their study of 703 undergraduates, Copenhaver and Grauerholz (1991) found that 14.7% of the women and 7.1% of the men reported dates in which the man had sexual intercourse with the woman against her wishes. The authors cite studies by Kanin and colleagues spanning 20 years in which 20.9% to 23.8% of college women reported experiencing forceful attempts at sexual intercourse while on dates during the past year (cited in Copenhauer & Grauerholz, 1991). Kanin further found that 25.5% of the unmarried male undergraduates surveyed reported making forceful attempts at sexual intercourse while on a date. Mills and Granoff (1992) found 28% of college women reported rape or attempted rape, and nearly 30% of men reported making advances after a woman refused. Among male college athletes, 27% admitted verbal coercion, 11% physical assault, and 4% admitted rape (Jackson, 1991).

PRESSURE, COERCION, AND CONSENT

Holland, Ramazanoglu, Sharpe, et al. (1991) delineate the continuum between consent and rape. They begin with verbal pressure comprising persuasion, where women consent to sex or unsafe sex that they don't want because of what they feel to be social pressures or the importance to them of their relationship or potential relationship with a man. In this situation, men did not need to take any decisive action to exert pressure for women to feel that they should submit. Verbal pressure from men may be experienced as coercive not directly because of the man's behavior but because of the woman's beliefs about the meanings of men's behavior and what would happen if intercourse were denied. In this case, women feel responsible for both creating and administering to men's arousal. Physical pressure characterized by intimidation was associated with situations where men interpreted a social relationship as entitling them to sex. Where women have been drunk, they are particularly unwilling to describe themselves as having been raped or physically forced into sex but rather that they must take responsibility because they had not been in condition to avoid unwanted sex. Women were sometimes unwilling to use the term *rape* when they felt they might somehow have been able to prevent or avoid the situation or when they had no basis of comparison for a consensual sexual experience. Even when a young woman was able to identify an incident as rape, Holland and colleagues found she might still blame herself.

NEGOTIATING CONSENT

The polarization between Gilbert and Paglia and feminist researchers, such as Russell and Koss (1992), prevents a discussion of the territory between rape and consent that may range from lack of explicit consent or encouragement to pressured consent, coercion, and force that stop short of rape. Sexual empowerment for both young women (and young men) could include a variety of choices: not engaging in sexual activity, not engaging in sexual activity without informed consent, getting partners to consent to safer practices, and negotiating sexual practices that are pleasurable to both partners (Holland, Ramazanoglu, Sharpe, et al., 1991).

Currently, negotiation is assumed to end when the woman agrees to have sex; it does not start at that point (Wight, 1992). For women to resist unwanted sex requires a model of a positive female sexuality that offers them a way of reflecting critically on their experiences of pressured sex (Fine, 1988; Holland, Ramazanoglu, Sharpe, et al., 1991). For men to resist coercion requires an egalitarian culture that promotes nonsexist and nonviolent rearing of male children (Sanday, 1990).

Both men and women must learn to enact ways of negotiating safe and pleasurable sex. Viewing empowerment as a contradictory and contested process, as Holland and colleagues do, is a point of departure for considering practical strategies for transforming pressured sexual relationships between women and men. I would criticize Paglia for her many public proclamations insisting that women must adapt their behavior to male expectations to avoid danger; in this way, women are yet again forced to accommodate their behavior to men's sexuality. On the other hand, I think Holland and others underestimate the extent to which women proceed with sex about which they might feel ambivalent, about which they have not yet decided, or that they may even not want. As Janet and Marianna told me, women sometimes have sex simply because they are afraid to be impolite or hurt their partners' feelings; they want to please their partners, avoid an argument, or because they don't know how to refuse or negotiate sex, having effectively internalized the feminine role. This makes the discussion on rape more ambiguous than the analysis of woman as victim would have it.

Young men today may not generally be as sexist as some feminist analyses assume, making refusing sex or asking for protection a less subversive act than Holland, Ramazanoglu, Sharpe, et al. (1991) and Fine (1988) would believe. Men are not the only ones invested in the status quo: It is difficult for women to overcome socialization and practice, even when they want to. To say that women are oppressed underestimates the complexity of the situation. This research contributes to the understanding of the construction of that complexity.

Notes

1. *Sassy*, Los Angeles: Peterson Publishing Company, October 1992.

2. *Tribadism* is one of the ways lesbians have sex, using legs—parallel to frottage among gay men.

3. I disagree with Camille Paglia, who refutes the idea of coercion, insists on ignoring the sanctions on women's sexuality, and further insists that adolescent women should have the same strength and assertiveness as she. Sex is more complicated than she makes it out to be.

4. Gilbert's views are restated in Gilbert, Muehlenhard, Highby, and Phelps (1997), with the rest disagreeing with him. Paglia was expressing her views in all the media she could access at the time (e.g., Paglia, 1990, 1993).

5. Dr. Russell's work includes *Men, Women and Rape; Femicide: The Politics of Woman Killing; Crimes Against Women: Proceedings of the International Tribunal; Making Violence Sexy: Feminist Views on Pornography; The Politics of Rape: The Victim's Perspective; Rape in Marriage; The Secret Trauma: Incest in the Lives of Girls and Women;* and *Sexual Exploitation: Rape, Child Sexual Abuse, and Workplace Harassment.*

6. Assessing the incidence of unreported rape is difficult because people may be seen at the women's clinic, regular medical clinics, social services, or the counseling and psychological service.

7

Sexual Negotiation Reconsidered

$\mathbf{T}$his study explored sexual negotiation among young adults. It primarily used focused interviews informed by questionnaires, university demographic and health service data, and informal interviews with university officials. The central portion of the research explored the themes that emerged from the in-depth interviews among 30 arts and science undergraduates of varying ethnic backgrounds and sexual orientations. Interviews focused on the normative influences of family, school, and friends regarding sexuality; understanding how relationships were negotiated and how trust and risk were constructed within relationships; how strategies for risk reduction, attitudes about HIV and testing, and contraceptive practices were managed differently by gender and sexual orientation; and what the barriers to safer sex were in various situations. In this chapter, I will consider the main findings of my research and their implications.

Normative Influences

I had expected family, school, and friends to be the major influences on sexual behavior among young adults. I encouraged participants to talk about their families' attitudes about sexuality, whether parents had talked about sex and to what extent. I attempted to probe for ethnic and social differences, but although participants were a diverse group, only Asians felt a specific influence of culture on sexuality. Individuals had been raised in a variety of family situations, from an inner-city student with a drug-addicted single parent to an affluent suburbanite. There were a couple of students whose parents had not finished primary school and a few whose parents had earned advanced degrees, yet there were few clues in content or style of interviews to distinguish among these differences. More salient than home or school, apparently, were the influences of friends, the social culture at university, and their interaction with the developmental tasks characteristic of the period between adolescence and adulthood.

SEX EDUCATION

Young adults are generally unprepared to communicate their sexual needs and desires by the time they reach university, even though most become sexually active in high school. According to the participants in this study, sex education before university was woefully inadequate. At home, it was usually limited to a description of reproduction or an ambiguous warning about being careful or using condoms. Most often, parents did not want to know about their children's sexual activities, but even where attempts were made at discussion, they were virtually always too little and too late. Perhaps if sexuality were discussed from an early age, it would be more useful when adolescents are ready to become sexually active. Clearly, parents cannot be counted on to prepare their children for healthy sex lives. Parents are often too ambivalent (at best) about their children having sex to encourage an open discussion of the experience. American culture may have something to learn from cultures that employ an aunt, uncle, or some other elder to instruct children about sexuality.

If we choose the school to fill that role, an unlikely possibility in the United States just now, consensus must be reached about what will be taught, for sex education in secondary school was also largely ineffective for these people. Students were dissatisfied with the quality and content of their sex education curricula prior to university. Both home and school instruction too often focused on reproductive function, seldom on the feelings involved in sexual awakening or how to handle sexual relationships in a positive way.

Young adults are thus left with little understanding of the intricacies of sexual relationships or experience talking about sex, which leaves them unprepared to negotiate either. Though most felt comfortable with their sexual activity, they had nonetheless simultaneously acquired notions of sex as taboo and stereotyped views of men as always ready and willing and women as responsible for controlling men's desires while suppressing their own. Participants in this study were usually ill-prepared for open communication with their sexual partners, with the result that early sexual experiences were unplanned and often unprotected.

On the other hand, a few participants reported learning a great deal from the university health education and sociology classes from which they were recruited. Some had learned to communicate more effectively in new sexual situations, others had incorporated spermicide, and still others commented on their increased tolerance for sexual diversity. Further research might examine whether they assimilated so much in university because the curriculum varied substantially from high school or because they were developmentally more prepared to attend to its content.

Formal sex education in the United States is in crisis, with little consensus about its essential elements. Debate continues on what should be taught and when to teach it. There is argument about whether or not "values" should be incorporated, as though education could ever be assumed to be value free. To be effective, sex education messages must be at once consistent and varied to reach everyone. Sex education must be ongoing because people may hear the same messages for years but not attend to them before they are ready. Sex education that acknowledges the complexity of situations that youth face and therefore presents safer sex as fun, empowering, and beneficial to relationships may be more acceptable to young people. School-based education is insufficient, however; HIV prevention should take place in the milieus in which people live and socialize and via meaningful networks of association.

Sex education must become more responsive to the real questions of adolescents and less subject to political wrangling. Education efforts must address more forcefully the canard that nice people don't get STDs, because the message has evidently not been incorporated, even among those who have contracted them.

Effective sex education must include information about intimacy, relationships, and communication in addition to details about sexuality. Young people need education that considers how emotions, sexual desire, and information interact in various situations to influence decision making and behavior. The impact of alcohol use in social and sexual situations, the role of casual relationships, and the potential hazards of parties should be discussed. Sex education that deconstructs sexuality can help young people understand the forces that influence their behavior.

This study supports the idea of the period between adolescence and adulthood as a developmental stage in its own right. As a developmental stage, it is marked by sexual experimentation and alcohol use. In the case of university students, the transition is negotiated primarily in the first year or two. Experimentation was an element of the experience of freedom but also served as part of identity formation, expressed through storytelling and impression management. The storytelling can be used as an exercise in intimacy among friends or more specifically as a way for young men to practice and maintain a particular masculine ideal (Holland et al., 1994).

I found participants extremely insightful about their situations and knowledgeable for the most part about STDs, but somehow, many were unable or unwilling to use that insight in sexual practice. The university setting supplies a fairly unstable, free environment in which many people at this stage were still subject to denial and wishful thinking regarding the potential consequences of their behavior. Further research would be needed to define whether these characteristics are unique to college students or whether they would apply to youth in other institutions, such as the military or the Peace Corps, or in noninstitutional situations, such as working or travelling directly after high school, or in other countries and cultures with discrete adolescent periods.

DRINKING AND SEXUAL EXPERIMENTATION

Drinking was a fundamental part of university social life; men especially felt social pressure to get drunk. Men used drinking to create a milieu for bonding, to facilitate expressiveness with each other, and for the pleasure of talking about their experiences while drinking. Fraternity parties were often mentioned as the site for drinking and "getting together" with someone, even among those who were not fraternity or sorority members. Neither co-ops nor off-campus housing featured in these accounts in the same way. According to responses on the Risk Assessment Questionnaire, students occasionally used pot, ecstasy, and other drugs; however, they did not emerge as important in the interviews and seemed not to serve the same social function as alcohol.

I had expected unsafe sexual practice to be a consequence of drinking; however, it turned out that both are elements of the same phenomenon, neither contingent on the other. People drank for fun and sometimes also to lubricate potential sexual situations. Drinking and not remembering sexual behavior was a recurrent theme, as was engaging in sexual behavior that one would not have done had one not been drinking. Coercive encounters occurred more frequently when partners had been drinking; the rules for sexual negotiation differed in this circumstance.

FRIENDS

Not surprisingly, friends were the most important influence in predicting whether an individual would practice safer sex. How and whether friends talked about sex and practiced safer sex were strong normative influences in predicting whether participants were having safer sex, a finding echoed by Romer et al. (1994) in their study of low-income young African American adolescents conducted during the same period as my own.

Men and women had different styles in talking about sex with their friends. Among men, feelings about relationships were often expressed through joking, although some men had learned to speak openly with one or two close friends. Both men and women felt they could be more frank with women: Discussions about sex among women were considerably more explicit than those among men, and women monitored their friends' behavior more closely than men did. Friends acted as an important source of information and support for both sexes, providing condoms, reassurance, a forum for advice, and a place to talk through problems. Men made themselves available to each other to recount their sexual experiences. They were willing to listen but didn't seem to find it morally appropriate to pressure each other to talk about sex or even to engage in safer sex as often as women did. Men might question a friend's unsafe sexual behavior but generally, they were nonjudgmental with each other.

Friends usually had similar sexual values and practices that they reinforced for each other. These friends might actively encourage or inhibit safer sex behavior; they might also monitor each other's behavior. Talking about sex enabled a forum for influence but was not the only way friends affected each other's behavior. Friends' behavior itself had an impact: Where friends practiced unsafe sex, requiring safer sex became difficult for an individual to imagine. In cases where an individual's values were dissonant with friends', a tension was created wherein they might try to influence each other or where one of them was independently trying to incorporate the values of the friends. Intervention on a group level may be one valuable approach where the norms of a group can be identified.

Experiential Responses to HIV and Safer Sex

One aim of this study was to explore the checks and balances that people use to evaluate risk and trust in developing relationships. This included eliciting information about HIV and other STDs; the intersection of safer sex and contraceptive practice; the processes of negotiation and profiles of change among individuals in a period of rapid change; and the means of communication, sources of support, and barriers to safer sex practices. The construction of risk was balanced between knowledge about HIV and a social climate that inconsistently supported safer sex practice. How risk was managed depended on the type of relationship anticipated and varied by sex and sexual orientation; however, risky behavior was uniformly denied or rationalized by everyone when it occurred.

THE CONSTRUCTION OF RISK

Risk was constructed in terms of both behavior and individuals. Participants had generally accurate information about transmission of HIV; however, two women felt that using a condom part way through or after having once engaged in unprotected intercourse with a given partner would be pointless. One gay man was not aware that insertive anal sex was a risky behavior. Several gay men mentioned avoiding fellatio if they had oral sores or had brushed their teeth, but did not seem to be aware of any possibility of transmission through healthy tissue. The gay men were certainly most aware of the reality of risk for HIV but there were no other defining characteristics that predicted how seriously an individual would take HIV. Most students accepted condoms for genital or anal intercourse as a fact of modern sexual life but not for oral sex. This is in no way surprising, for the need for condoms for fellatio is contested even (or especially) in gay communities. It is a difference in the social construction of risk I have noticed between the United States and Australia. Where condom use has been fairly commonly promoted as a risk-reduction strategy for fellatio among gay men in the United States, it appears generally regarded as unnecessary in Australia and barely features in the social discourse, which currently stresses open communication and testing as a precaution.[1] Protecting themselves from other STDs was not usually taken into consideration, seldom arising as an issue even among those who had previously contracted one.

MANAGING RISK

Young people use a variety of strategies to manage risk, from considering a partner's background, life situation, and knowledge about HIV to attempting to minimize their exposure to seminal and vaginal fluids. However, their strategies had limits: no one, regardless of sexual orientation, consistently used barrier methods for oral sex, although they tried to reduce their risk by using withdrawal for fellatio. Furthermore, strategies may not be employed uniformly: Resolve failed in the presence of a highly desirable partner, when aroused, and especially when drinking. Many people mentioned engaging in sex while drinking that otherwise would not have occurred. Other factors that predicted unsafe sex included those that related to the difficulty of communication about sex between partners, poor judgment about the risk involved in a behavior or situation, ambivalence about having sex, and the inability to consider alternatives to intercourse. Encouraging a diverse repertoire of sexual behaviors throughout the lifespan may help elevate less risky sexual behavior to the status of "real" sex, extending protection and still offering satisfaction.

Risk for pregnancy was distinguished from risk for HIV, although using condoms to address the risks simultaneously was not uncommon. The contraceptive landscape was simple for participants, either condoms or oral contraceptives: Diaphragm use was mentioned by only one person, no one mentioned caps, IUDs, or rarely even foam or gel. Sexual practice is equally simply articulated: for heterosexuals, *sex* was defined as genital intercourse, oral sex served only as occasional foreplay; even gay men were largely limited to oral or anal intercourse. Specific lesbian sexual practices were not common enough to discuss here.

Testing for HIV antibodies before beginning a new sexual relationship proved to be a far less important strategy than I had expected, seldom employed or considered by the heterosexual men. Gay men tested more routinely and more often thought about repeat testing than other participants. Women considered testing more often than straight men because they were accustomed to the linking of sexuality with medical practice. Because they are always conscious of the risk for pregnancy and may have had experience with tests for pregnancy or STDs or pelvic exams for contraception, managing risk medically seemed reasonable to them in a heterosexual context. There was more ambivalence about testing than I had expected, expressed mainly through procrastination.

Risk was perceived differently by men and women. Men, regardless of sexual orientation, tended not to question their partners about their sexual histories, using appearance more often than women to evaluate a potential partner and worrying about their risk of exposure after a sexual encounter. They relied more on information about a potential partner's background and lifestyle than on actual questioning about sexual history or evidence from STD test results. Lowy and Ross (1994) found this among gay men in Australia, suggesting a strongly gender-related strategy.

CONSTRUCTING HIV: DISTANCE, DISSONANCE, AND RISK

People handled dissonance about their behavior by creating distance. They reduced the import of their behavior by denying its risk, by comparing it to behavior they considered riskier, or simply by depersonalizing their situation. When considering risk for HIV as too threatening or too remote, individuals may focus instead on contraceptive issues or more common STDs. If risk then is assessed in terms of mutual trust and degree of intimacy in the relationship, it is applied only to the extent that accurate information about transmission is known, believed, and personalized. No matter how much education is provided or how relevant it is, we should probably accept that there will remain a proportion of people such as Ann and George who simply will not relate risk to themselves. As noted previously, most participants presented their behavior as calculated in terms of risk and benefits. Several participants, notably Wheeler and Hanan, didn't perceive their potential risks because they used what they saw as protection for the most part, exemplifying the case of behavior in conflict with a self-concept as scrupulously careful and underscoring the argument that risk is subjectively and not objectively constructed.

One third of the interview participants had known someone who was HIV+, but none mentioned it as a salient influence on their behavior. For those who took HIV seriously, precautionary behavior seemed more often to be part of an impression of societal change. The concept of being HIV+ evoked varying reactions. Some women expressed concern for their partners and families over themselves. For other participants, the notion of justice was elicited, the idea that if one found oneself HIV+, the status would have been deserved because of untoward behavior.

Categories of Relationships: Implications for Protection

Relationships evolved as either casual or romantic, with partners beginning as strangers or friends, each form with its own contraceptive and protective practices that could best be understood in the context of the given relationship. Styles in evaluating risk and managing safer sex were predicted more often by gender than sexual orientation. Regardless of the type of relationship, open communication remained difficult for young adults of all sexual orientations, making trust the cornerstone of assessing risk. Negotiating sex and consistently maintaining safer sex practice remained a challenge, although gay and bisexual participants had made more progress in this arena than heterosexuals.

COMMUNICATION AND PROTECTION IN
CASUAL AND ROMANTIC RELATIONSHIPS

Casual relationships began between people who had just met or between acquaintances. In these types of relationships, appearance was often used to assess a potential partner's risk, especially by men. Partners who didn't know each other well might talk about their previous relationships as a way of becoming more intimate and assessing each other's risk simultaneously. How individuals regarded and used condoms proved to be embedded in a set of personal attitudes that differed by context of relationship. In casual relationships, condoms were usually used until or unless the relationship became more committed. Commitment was signalled by a discussion about the progress and future of the relationship and could occur as quickly as 3 weeks on. If partners decided not to make a commitment at that point, both recognized the need for continued protection; conversely, making a promise of exclusivity involved a shift to a romantic relationship that implied safety and trust. Where sexual encounters occurred between heterosexual friends, condoms were less likely to be used because the man often knew beforehand that the woman was on the pill, because the partner was trusted by virtue of being a friend, and because the partners had usually been drinking.

Among participants who began in a romantic dating relationship, the couple dated for what they considered "a long time," variously between 3 months and a year, before engaging in intercourse. For heterosexuals, the romantic relationship was prototypical of women's responsibility to control the progression of sexual activity. Men attempted to bring the sexual activity to the next level; women felt required to control them. Once the relationship included regular sexual activity, however, the woman was often an equal participant in initiating and sustaining an encounter. Because trust was established in what partners assumed to be a monogamous relationship before sexual activity occurred, oral contraceptives might be used either instead of or after a short period of condom use. Before going on the pill, women often wanted to know officially whether they were in a committed relationship, sometimes symbolized by HIV testing.

Women tended to evaluate risk in terms of the type of relationship more often than men (i.e., whether the encounter would be casual or was part of a romantic relationship). In heterosexual encounters, they made decisions similarly about specific sexual acts within the context of the type of relationship in which they were involved; for example, they usually engaged in fellatio only with partners to whom they felt committed. If they believed they were in a committed relationship, they trusted their partner and might therefore be willing to forgo condoms in what they presumed was a monogamous relationship. Regarding more casual encounters, women were aware that men tended not to consider risk before a sexual encounter; their reactions ranged from acceptance to bitterness about what they perceived as men's lack of concern. On the other hand, men were aware that women were concerned with protecting their reputations, supporting Wight's (1992) explanation that lack of discussion and acknowledgment occur because it is important to maintain ambiguity in case one of the partners decides not to continue.

Casual relationships may be labelled in misleading ways by couples to protect the reputation or identity of a partner. Such situations may engender risk—for example, where a woman is concerned about her reputation, they might need to maintain the pretense that casual encounters are really relationships. This means pretending to trust the partner, which may mean not using or asking to use condoms or not questioning a partner's sexual history. Partners may subscribe to an ideology of romance while simultaneously engaging in casual encounters, making it difficult to behave as though they believe their behaviors were risky. Although lesbian relationships were not common enough to generalize about, women spoke of both trusting their female partners more and feeling less at risk from them.

BALANCING RISK AND REPUTATION

Both men and women were aware that women risked their reputations by acknowledging their sexual desires. Women found it difficult to tell their partners they wanted sex because of what they had been taught about the physical and emotional risks involved and the messages they had received about appropriate behavior for young women. A heterosexual woman's reputation often had more to do with the extent to which her friends were aware of her behavior than the objective number of men with whom she had been involved. When a woman experimented sexually, her friends' reactions ranged from pressure to have many partners to sanctions against having too many. The double standard remains: epithets that describe women who have many partners are universally disparaging, whereas those that describe men are rather laudatory. Women still set the pace for sexual intimacy because they worry about their reputations; men are nonetheless expected to be prepared to produce condoms at the appropriate moment, making open communication about safer sex difficult.

THE CONSTRUCTION OF TRUST

The low seroprevalence of HIV among college students at this time makes risk a difficult question to resolve where people don't perceive themselves as in a life-threatening situation—partly for good reason. Conceptions of trust varied from accepting someone's word about safety to being perceived a caring partner if transmission of HIV was always assumed to be a possibility.

HIV has made the issue of trust in sexual relationships a potential question of life and death. Where betrayal formerly meant dealing with the feelings associated with a partner's nonmonogamy, the implications have now become more serious. Although fidelity in American culture is normally constructed as synonymous with monogamy, it was not defined as such for everyone. There was room for some in the construction of trust to include safer sex outside relationships, informing partners of outside relationships, being honest with each other. To the degree that a partner's word was insufficient as the basis of trust, other means of establishing confidence included getting tested for HIV individually, together, regularly, or both of the last two; checking one's perception of a partner with friends; and having condoms available and always using them. Each method of establishing confidence was but a piece of a whole, illusory by itself.

NEGOTIATING SAFER SEX

Negotiating for safer sex contained elements of impression management, required assertiveness, and took constant effort even for those who had made the most progress in incorporating it. For my study participants, *safer sex* had come to be defined as condom use for vaginal or anal intercourse, with little imagination left over to attempt spermicide, barriers for oral sex, or alternative forms of sexual expression. Although many individuals had learned to use condoms consistently for intercourse, certainly a sign of progress, only one had never lapsed, and none was using them on more than an experimental basis for oral sex; furthermore, no one mentioned having reservations about the efficacy of condoms.

Participants varied widely in the amount of thought and practice they had put into negotiating sexual relationships. Those who were not heterosexual had considered the issues of safer sex in more depth and more often attempted creative change. That gay men should have done so was certainly not surprising; more surprising was that the bisexual women in this study had also attempted changes that heterosexuals had not. Only the gay men and bisexual women had used gloves, condoms, or dental dams for oral sex, sporadically even then. In spite of the difficulty of negotiation, several participants were certain they would not engage in intercourse without condoms under any circumstance. Some viewed safer sex as fun or empowering, because it forced them to communicate more openly, to be more creative in the approach to sex, and to be more responsible for their behavior. Presenting safer sex as fun or empowering could be a key indicator in promoting its discussion and practice.

For those who practiced them, safer sex behaviors were not always easy to incorporate or maintain and sometimes needed reevaluation or renegotiation over time. Even talking about safer sex or sexual histories with a prospective or new partner could be difficult because of what such discussions implied about trust. When sex is used to create intimacy, it is difficult to discuss its implications. Talking about sex may be interpreted as a sexual act itself, so engaging in sex may be less revealing in some respects than talking about it. However, a safer sex discussion may be necessary before the intent to engage in sex has been clearly signalled. A relationship may have been established without prior discussion and raising the topic later implies a lack of trust. For these reasons, condoms were seldom discussed before they were needed; rather, the discussion often remained general and focused on family and past relationship patterns instead of specific details of sexual history. Additional behavior changes were incorporated sequentially and not simultaneously, suggesting that mastery of safer sex is a complicated process that occurs over time.

Conclusions, Implications, and Recommendations

Practicing safer sex involves an intricate process of sexual negotiation: How sex is negotiated depends on the construction of risk
and trust between partners, which varies by the type of relationship
or sexual encounter being contemplated. Among young adults, the
necessity for safer sex comes precisely at a time of experimentation
with alcohol and sex that makes its negotiation problematic. To be
effective, HIV prevention programming must take these dynamics
into account.

This study examined the construction of trust and risk among
young adults. How do people deal with trust in the context of the
possibility of contracting a fatal illness? How do they perceive their
responsibility; can they even perceive themselves as a potential risk
to someone else? Once people are aware of the risks of HIV, what are
the circumstances that allow them to trust? In the standard progression
of romantic relationships, after trust has been established, condoms
are no longer needed. Yet trust is defined in contradistinction not only
to risk but to betrayal. Evidence of a partner's nonmonogamy, an
STD, pregnancy, or even gaining new health information may alter
the checks and balances of risk assessment. When a person learns that
a partner has been nonmonogamous or unsafe with someone else, it
causes a re-evaluation of what would be required to trust in the future. These are the types of traumatic incidents that may cause people
to change their ideas about trust, their attitudes and practices. A challenge for intervention is to help people protect themselves in the
absence of betrayal, particularly in the early stages of a relationship
where a partner's trustworthiness may not have been established.

Intervention on a group level might be useful where the norms of
the group can be identified; the health promotion outreach that already takes place in the university dormitories might be more effectively extended to other arenas, such as co-ops and fraternities. Although the fraternities currently have health workers who have safer
sex material and condoms available, the pressure against trying to
influence friends' behavior in fraternities must be reckoned with to
make their work more effective. Peggy Reeves Sanday (1990) views
fraternities themselves as ritual sites for coercive sexual behavior
because of the male bonding function they serve. Copenhaver and
Grauerholz (1991) suggest institutional change, including mandatory acquaintance rape programming for fraternity members, now
available on few campuses, with a university "watchperson" as-
signed to monitor behavior. Mandatory peer education programs

and workshops could extend to related issues, such as safe alcohol use, gender roles, and safer sex. Perhaps these efforts could cause new cohorts of fraternity members to question the acceptability of negative or unhealthy behaviors that are currently supported by fraternity culture. Friendship networks could provide an important intervention point for AIDS education, especially where educators use different approaches to reach men and women. Only one person mentioned UC Berkeley's peer educators; it might be useful to evaluate the effectiveness of such programs in the various settings in which they occur.

RESEARCH ON HIV TESTING

Research focusing on the testing experience could clarify whether young peoples' procrastination regarding testing was truly due to inconvenience and organization or to the complex of emotions surrounding the testing experience. Encouraging a general strategy of testing between partners and waiting for test results before beginning sexual activity could be encouraged as a safer sex tool for those who are serially monogamous with breaks in between relationships. If convenience were truly the barrier, confidential or anonymous testing, education, and counselling could be offered at dorms and fraternities, provided a positive foundation were laid for the perception of testing as a strategy. Among relatively low-risk university students, accessible testing offers a point of entry for counselling and education that can help them consider their behaviors in light of more common threats, such as other sexually transmissible diseases and the effects of alcohol or recreational drugs on their ability to negotiate the sex they want.

RESEARCH AMONG SPECIFIC POPULATIONS:
ETHNICITY, CLASS, SEXUAL ORIENTATION, AND GENDER

More research is needed on ethnicity, class, and the change process, especially among nonstudent groups of the same age. Sexual communication itself needs further study, particularly among heterosexual men and lesbians. Understanding the limitations of the present state of sexual research will help to further define the discourse on sexual negotiation. Because my study found ethnically specific attitudes and behavior among only Asian students, further study focusing more on ethnicity would be useful, especially by non-White researchers. There were unquestionably class differences among the participants; several mentioned being raised in inner-city

Los Angeles, some by single parents, but the relationship of such differences to sexual negotiation was difficult to distinguish among university students.

I might speculate briefly at the dearth of lesbian participants. Sexuality in general is processual for youth. Bisexuality seemed to be more of a phase for men than for women; for men, coming to university gave them the opportunity to realize their homosexuality. Women may be more bisexual than men or may reach their endpoint in defining sexual orientation at a later age than men, as gender role socialization may prevent women from acting on their lesbian attractions where they have been accustomed to a sexuality that is more often responsive than active. It may also take longer for women to come out because they may then also need to readjust gender-socialized expectations about career, family, and supporting themselves.

As a consequence of heterosexual women's inability to articulate their desire, men can hope for sex, but neither men nor women plan for it realistically. This poses a problem for the promotion and practice of safer sex. As long as sexual relationships are defined by men pressuring and women resisting, open discussion about safer sex and alternative sexual expression will remain difficult. When women can acknowledge their desire for sex and men do not need to pressure or second-guess them, both sexes should be able to negotiate more openly about safer sex and sexual boundaries. On this count, Holland et al. (1994) recommend a gendered dimension in the development of policy and practice for HIV and AIDS prevention.

Although more is known about heterosexual women's sexuality than perhaps any other group's, there is little detailed knowledge about the unique challenges of sexual communication among other categories of individuals.[2] Men's discourse on sex seemed opaque; further research should specifically explore men's styles of communication and how they support and influence each other. Collaborative approaches might be most effective: Because both men and women find it easier to confide in women, female researchers may be more appropriate for obtaining sensitive information. However, it is essential that male researchers participate in interpreting results and probably also in doing outreach to men. The Heterosexual Men's Project of Family Planning New South Wales in Sydney[3] has used a male project worker and the results of qualitative research to reach and involve men. The project attempts to integrate perceptions of risk for HIV with other STDs, recognizing the need for clinical and educational services specific to men. Further valuable research among men could include qualitative study with men identified as coercive, if they could feel safe enough to explore and explain their thoughts and behaviors. Feminists, myself included, believe that men fundamentally know when they are behaving coercively; understanding just how they interpret such behavior for themselves offers material for intervention. Heterosexual men, bisexual women and men, gay and lesbian youth, and young people whose sexual orientation may be in transition all warrant further in-depth study. Although this work contributes to the extension of knowledge about sexuality and sexual communication among youth of both sexes and various sexual orientations, more remains to be done.

CONTINUING ISSUES IN THE STUDY OF SEXUALITY

It is difficult to deconstruct sexuality from within one's own culture: how does one write about sex without using the same heuristic terms that one criticizes as imprecise? Sexual behavior, sexual orientation, and gender role are all multidimensional, a concept that is almost impossible to grasp in Western culture.[4] There are both theoretical and practical implications for these difficulties: how do we design prevention without language? Furthermore, if we are prevented by the nonsecular moralists from doing sex surveys and sex education, how do we suggest alternatives to risky sex while keeping them defined as *sex* so that people still feel like the behavior is legitimate, that they're having fun, that it counts? An expanded definition of safer sex will go beyond the use of condoms to include analyses of trust in relationships, sexual identity as process, the risky self, STDs, gendered ideologies of sexuality and violence, the effect of alcohol on sexual negotiation, and the generation of discursive resources among heterosexuals with which to mobilize safer sex.

Epilogue: The Cultural Representation of HIV and Interactionist Understanding

As we examine personal sexual interaction, the cultural representations of sexuality and HIV can be examined to inform individual sense-making. Between the time this research was undertaken in 1992-1993 and the time I am revising it in the latter half of 1996, public discourse on HIV has changed it from an indiscriminate menace to young and old alike to a disease of disadvantage. What has changed in 3 years? The threat-to-the-general-population-that-never-was has largely dissolved. But for a week at the 11th International Conference on AIDS in July, media coverage has turned elsewhere. Discussion of

AIDS in the Usenet discussion group *sci.med.aids* is a shadow of its former self. Rates of gonorrhea and chlamydia have declined among White youth and continue to rise among Black youth. Most people in the world with HIV are heterosexual, live in poor countries, and will never have access to expensive vaccines or combination therapies—just as they were in 1993. The majority of new cases of HIV infection in rich countries also tends to be among disadvantaged people: intravenous drug users and their sexual partners, disproportionate numbers of African Americans and Hispanics in the United States, young gay men, especially men of color. Prevalence trends have not changed much in that time, but public perception has. An interactionist perspective can keep AIDS on the agenda as a global issue, preventing it from returning full circle to a disease of the Other.

Notes

1. This is not meant to imply that condoms are actually *used* more for oral sex in America, only that they are part of the public discourse in gay communities and among sexual health service providers. Nor do I mean to imply that condoms are never mentioned or recommended by their Australian counterparts, but they have not been part of AIDS campaigns, and oral sex is presented as a low-risk behavior for gay men.

2. Except for certain high risk youth: Some work has been done with runaway youth and youth living in shelters, groups homes, or detention centers.

3. This agency's address is Family Planning NSW Ltd., 328-336 Liverpool Road, Ashfield 2131, Australia; fax: 61 2 9716 6164, phone: 61 2 9716 6099.

4. Although those involved in AIDS prevention are attempting expansive and creative definitions, it is hard to imagine such terms as *men who have sex with men* or *MSM* gaining common currency outside of academic and health circles.

Appendix: Methodological Procedures and Issues

Rapport and the Researcher as Research Instrument

Because of my 17 years of experience in counselling and reproductive health, I was comfortable and familiar with eliciting sensitive information about sexuality. Both men and women were almost uniformly forthcoming. Several men mentioned that they could more easily talk intimately about sex with their female friends, and I assumed their frankness extended to me in the same way. Because I was mostly concerned with the construction of relationships, interviews normally did not focus on specific sexual acts. In the first interview, I was rather tentative, uncertain of what would be prying, what might make Sarita comfortable, how much I could ask about sex as opposed to the more general topic of relationships. I learned that most of the people who signed up had a lot to say and were willing to disclose intimate details. Only one participant, Theresa, had so few opinions and so little affect that I did not transcribe the interview. I made notes about it when I got home and listened to the tape again when I began writing. She was included in the analysis as far as possible, but the reader will notice very little contribution from her in the preceding chapters. I wondered whether she had little to say because she was sexually inexperienced, but another student was also a virgin yet had a good deal to say.

Beginning with the ninth participant, I had students complete the Bem Sex Role Inventory (BSRI) (Bem, 1977, 1981) and the Risk Assessment Questionnaire (RAQ) before the interview. This had the result of ice breaking and priming them; they talked about intimate topics more readily; I found I needed to spend less time opening them up. Where possible, I glanced at their RAQ before the interview; knowing their responses helped direct some of the questions. Before that point, when I'd look at it after the interview, I'd see responses that I might have explored in the interview had I been aware of them. For example, noting that a participant scored herself as somewhat bisexual gave me a chance to address this topic, opening up some of her feelings about gender relations.

Although I perceived no difficulty in eliciting very intimate information, I still wondered about ways in which I or the interview situation may have biased the data collection. Most of the time, interviews were interesting and enjoyable, but there were times that I felt frustrated and even bored. I believe I managed to appear nonjudgmental when George recounted his extremely sexist opinions and Ann her elaborate rationalizations (and in a perverse way, these characteristics made them among the most interesting of the interviews), the evidence being the quality of information I received from them. I don't know what I could have done to get Theresa or Karen to open up more: I was aware of my moods going into interviews and adjusted accordingly, they seemed simply not to have a great deal to say. Joanna, who was Karen's flatmate, was interviewed directly after Karen, and she seemed to be more forthcoming, even though I was tired by then. In my analysis, I have tried to be aware of any gender bias in interpreting men's realities and have had some helpful comments from a male colleague who pointed out that just because men do things differently than women doesn't make them less evolved.

Data Collection Procedures

To distinguish results, *participants* refers to those who gave interviews and also completed questionnaires, *respondents* to members of any of the three classes who completed only the RAQ.

INTERVIEW PARTICIPANTS

Study participants were UC Berkeley undergraduates: interviewees were recruited from a lower-division introductory health education class and a sociology of sexuality class. Recruitment of volunteers for interviews occurred in two phases: in October 1992, I visited the health education class to recruit volunteers for interviews. Sign-up sheets were passed around during the lecture; 45 students volunteered, with whom 19 interviews were arranged between November and August.

Only 6.2% of RAQ respondents in the first class and 5% in the second class had had "significant gay or lesbian attraction or experience," finally yielding only 2 interviews of the 19 from this class. Sampling was theoretically driven by sex, academic level, ethnicity, and sexual orientation. Choices of informants and questions were shaped more by conceptual questions than a desire for representativeness, hence the oversampling of gay and bisexual participants: Because I considered it important to combine sexualities in one study, I approached the visiting professor teaching Sociology of Sexual Diversity to recruit more volunteers for interviews. Recruitment in this second phase was successful; 36 additional people signed up.

Among interview participants from all groups, no women classified themselves as primarily or exclusively lesbian. One third of all interview participants considered themselves bisexual or gay. Although I might have expected a selection bias by virtue of the course topics, individuals proved demographically representative; both interview participants and survey respondents were representative of arts and science students on the Berkeley campus, though possibly not of undergraduates as a whole (i.e., not including engineering or business school students, for example).

I presented myself to all classes as a doctoral candidate doing dissertation research on relationships. The respective professors encouraged students to cooperate as a civic action. I estimated that the time required for the interview and completion of two questionnaires would be about 2 hours. I downplayed the fact that participants would be compensated monetarily,[1] and indeed, most were surprised when I offered them money at the end. Most were given $15 at the end of interviews; one or two refused payment. Only one person ever asked about money when I phoned to arrange an interview; he didn't make an appointment. Most were happy to cooperate, even when months had elapsed after recruitment. I began interviews with upper-division students because I thought they might have a broader perspective on their university careers that would inform interviews with younger participants.

RAQ RESPONDENTS

The instructor of the health education class from which I recruited interview participants later agreed to have the RAQ distributed to discussion sections. Questionnaires were placed in large envelopes, with the following instructions for the tutorial section leader to read aloud:

> These forms are part of Dana Lear's dissertation research on how young adults form relationships. They are meant to complement qualitative interviews by giving me an idea of background variables of young women and men today. They are designed to be anonymous and are completely voluntary. They are not related to and will have no effect on your course grade, nor will they be seen by [the instructor]. Please do not discuss your answers with your classmates until they have all been collected—then feel free to use them as a springboard for discussion.

Section leaders were further requested to complete the cover sheet with the number of students registered in the section, the number present on that day, and the date. They were asked to distribute and collect the questionnaires in one session, seal the envelope, and return it to the instructor. Of the 78 students present in section, 67 completed questionnaires, a return rate of 85.9%. Among those sections, there were 97 students registered; I was told that athletes tended to be nonattenders, but I am not aware of any other irregularities. Athletes were a group that was not well-represented, but, like fraternity members, I suspect they are a group worthy of further research and intervention along the lines of Peggy Reeves Sanday's (1990) *Fraternity Gang Rape*, given both groups' reputations among their peers. Rick, the football player, was one man who talked about the difference in public and private discourse about sex, and this would be one issue to explore further among athletes. The main obstacle to good return was a graduate student strike during the distribution period, with the result that three sections did not meet; some of the missing students in the remaining classes may have stayed away in sympathy.

Additional surveys were distributed to a second health education class the following semester. These were distributed at the door on the day of a test review session, 45 of approximately 60 present, or approximately 75%, responded. Interview volunteers were not recruited at this class. A third set of RAQs was distributed at the sociology class, from which additional interviewees were solicited. Unfortunately, this professor refused to have it distributed during class; instead, he invited students to pick up a survey on the way out and return it next class; thus, only 17 of among approximately 100 students returned surveys.

Data Management, Coding, and Analysis

DATA MANAGEMENT: INTERVIEWS

Interviews were tape recorded and transcribed in their entirety, save one that had yielded very little useful information. Initial transcription was done to computer disk by a professional, after which I listened to each tape to correct errors and complete omissions, backed up disks, and printed a hard copy. Each tape took about 3 hours to verify after transcription. I listened to the tapes again just before beginning the writing, to ensure my coding had been true to the material and to refresh the experience of the interviews. These transcriptions were then saved as text files and coded in Hyper-RESEARCH[tm] for the Macintosh.

HyperRESEARCH[tm] is a HyperCard-based application that allows for qualitative and quantitative analysis of textual material through the following functions: coding of text, retrieval of coded materials, testing propositions through the use of Boolean searches, and hypothesis testing. Textual passages can be multiply coded and codes can be deleted, copied, and renamed (Hesse-Biber, Dupuis, & Kinder, 1991). It claims to be useful in hypothesis formation and testing, but I could not make it work for this purpose.

CODING AND DATA ANALYSIS

Initial coding was very close to the text, resulting at one point in 273 microcodes. As theory developed, I reviewed coded interviews to verify their completeness and accuracy, but it wasn't generally necessary to recode entire interviews once new codes arose. The resulting HyperRESEARCH[tm] report by case, code frequency, and text reference came to 250 single-spaced pages. From these codes, analysis began of the 175 microcodes that had emerged as most theoretically relevant (i.e., relating specifically to alcohol use, safe sex strategies and impediments, reference groups, trust and risk construction, sexual communication). Topics that I thought might be important but proved not to be salient (e.g., religiosity) were discarded. Microcodes were cleaned up, with duplicates and redundancies eliminated and codes refined. From these codes, I developed categories about the data, for example, defining the difference between low-probability or high-probability condom users or the influence of friends and family. It is from these codes that the three main categories of (a) normative influences, (b) negotiating relationships, and (c) negotiating sex emerged with their underlying themes, which are discussed in Chapters 3 through 6.

The Risk Assessment Questionnaire (RAQ)

To establish a baseline for evidence of unprotected sex, I analyzed UC Berkeley UHS statistics for STD and pregnancy testing for the 2 years prior to my research. These figures confirmed the UHS Health Promotion staff's estimates that approximately 25% of students contract STDs during their undergraduate careers. I spoke to the UC Police and the Health Promotion Unit regarding rape statistics and obtained demographic data from the Office of Student Research to assess representativeness of my sample on the basis of age, ethnicity, academic level, and sex. Students completing the questionnaire reflected undergraduate arts and sciences students on campus.

I designed the RAQ to gain demographic and sexual history information on the health and sexuality classes as a group. To avoid making students anxious about their answers, the RAQ was labelled simply "Assessment Questionnaire." In addition to general demographic information, I was interested in relationship and sexual histories and whether a history of child sexual abuse or intrarelationship violence might have any effect on sexual behavior. The RAQ was meant to both complement and theoretically inform the qualitative interviews; it was administered to interview participants and anonymously to three undergraduate classes. Parts of the questionnaire were analyzed using descriptive statistics; the open-ended questions were coded and analyzed for themes in a way similar to the interviews. Because it was meant for my own personal use along with the interviews and not as a primary method on its own, the questionnaire was not tested for validity and reliability.

The RAQ is a three-page form that takes 10 to 15 minutes to complete. Questions designed to provide information on family include ethnic background, where the person was raised, religious observance, age of parents (to provide insight on parents' sexual generation), and parents' level of education (for information on socioeconomic status and perhaps social attitudes). I asked about drinking and recreational drug use, fraternity membership, history of sexual abuse, past and present sexual orientation, relationship history, history of coercive sex and relationship violence, pregnancy and STD history, safer sex practices, and acquaintance with an HIV+ person.

The RAQ evolved in its early stages: After the first interview, I added two questions about the role of alcohol or recreational drugs in sexual encounters; this revised form was used in further interviews and in the first distribution of the form in December 1992. As a result of ambiguous responses to the questions on sexual coercion, I added two questions about perpetration of intrarelationship violence. The ambiguity was indicated by an affirmative response in the relationship matrix indicating coercive sexual experience but negative response to the item asking whether a partner had pressured, coerced, or forced sexual acts. The latter version was used in subsequent classes and interviews in the spring and summer of 1993. The relationship matrix was adapted from that used in the Women Risk and AIDS Project questionnaire (Holland, Ramazanoglu, Scott, et al., 1991; Holland, Ramazanoglu, Sharpe, et al., 1991); my respondents found it fairly confusing, though it still yielded usable information about numbers of sexual partners.

The RAQ was used to gather demographic and other background data to inform interviews and provide baseline information on sexual experiences common to university youth. For example, it informed interviews with respect to sexuality as process, the importance of drinking, the discrepancy between conceptions of safer sex and actual safer sex practice, and the lack of salience of acquaintance with an HIV+ person. The only anomaly I noticed on the RAQ was a low proportion of drinkers, given the large role alcohol played in the interview stories. Closed-ended items were analyzed separately for class respondents and interview participants using StatView SE+Graphics.

SEX, RACE, AND CLASS

The interview participants in this study were truly a diverse group. There were 16 women and 14 men (57:43). The vast majority, 87%, applied to Berkeley as California residents. Two thirds grew up in Southern California, and of those, half came from Los Angeles. Reflecting the changing face of California, more than half had at least one parent born outside of the United States. Four were themselves foreign-born, but only three were even partly foreign-raised. The ethnic and age distribution were compared to the class members who completed questionnaires and to the campus letters and science undergraduates.

The largest proportion of participants was Caucasian, followed by Asian, African American, and Latino. Students with one Latino parent and one of European origin were classified as Latino, making the proportion of Latino students in this sample unusual by campus standards. According to the Office of Student Research, they classify multicultural students similarly, using the less common ethnicity as the identifier, even if it is not the predominant one (see Table A1).

The racial distribution of interview participants is compared with questionnaire respondents and letters and science undergraduates in Table A2.

Several participants mentioned growing up in inner-city Los Angeles, but it was difficult from the interviews to ascertain any effects of social class on individuals' attitudes or behavior. Mother's level of education ranged from 5th grade to PhD; the two mothers with primary school education were both Mexican-born; another student had a Mexican-born mother with college education.

The average age of members of this sample was 20.7 years, matching the campus undergraduate average of 20.8 years. Class standing was heavily weighted toward upper class because I felt that juniors and seniors would be better able to reflect on the college years. The age distribution is shown in Table A3.

SEXUALITY

The average age of sexual debut was 16.6 years, older than Trocki's 1992 sample of the neighboring East Bay county but similar to the national average and the age cited by Bienenstock and Epstein (1979), who found a mean age of 16.2 to 16.5 between 1971 and 1976. Wyatt (1989) found that 98% of Caucasian and African American women had debuted by the age of 20 years, I found 90% had by the age of 19 years. Among my interview participants, one man and one woman, both heterosexual, had not yet engaged in genital intercourse, although the man had engaged in oral-genital sex. The age of sexual debut by race in descending order was African American, 17.75 years; Asian, 17.5; Latino, 16.6; and Caucasian, 15.6. Among RAQ respondents, age of sexual debut among women was 16.89 years among women and 16.58 years among men, with a median age of 17 for both sexes, compared to a national average of 16 and Trocki's average of 15.

Among interviewees, 16.7% had contracted an STD at some point, but it is impossible to say whether they would equal the campus average of 25% by the time they all graduated. Their presumed

Table A1 Selected Demographic Characteristics of Interview Participants

Name	Year in School	Sexual Orientation	Age	Age of Sexual Debut	Ethnic Origin	U.S.-Born	Where Raised	Mother, Father U.S.-Born	Mother's Education
1. Sarita	4	1	21	17	India	Yes	Northern California	No	MS degree
2. Rita	4	1	22	18	China-Japan	No	Southern California	No	BA degree
3. Janice	4	2	21	16	Europe	Yes	Los Angeles	Yes, No	High School
4. George	4	1	21	14	England	Yes	Nevada	Yes	BA degree
5. Vicky	4	1	21	18	China	Yes	Northern California	No	n/a
6. Karen	3	1	20	15	England	Yes	South Bay (Northern California)	Yes	n/a
7. Joanna	3	2	20	16	Europe	Yes	Southern California	Yes	n/a
8. Sonia	3	2	21	18	Nicaragua	No	Northern California, Nicaragua	No	Some college
9. Charlie	2	2	19	17	China	Yes	New York	No	College
10. Hanan	2	1	20	18	Egypt-Ethiopia	Yes	Los Angeles	No	BS degree
11. Lauren	2	1	19	15	England	Yes	Los Angeles	No	High school
12. Denise	4	4	22	13	Mexico-Europe	Yes	Southern California	No, Yes	MA degree
13. Theresa	4	1	22	—	Peru-Italy	Yes	Los Angeles	No, Yes	Some college
14. Dave	3	7	19	17	China	No	Taiwan	No	College
15. Eric	1	1	18	—	Europe	Yes	Oregon	Yes	MA degree
16. Rick	1	1	18	16	Mexico	Yes	Southern California	Yes	Jr. college
17. Ginger	2	4	20	18	China-Hong Kong	Yes	Southern California	No	High school
18. Shawn	3	1	20	15	Europe	Yes	Los Angeles	Yes	MA degree

19. Donald	1	6	19	17	Africa-America	Yes	Los Angeles	Yes	PhD degree
20. Raphael	5	5	22	19	Mexico-Europe	Yes	East Bay (Northern California)	Yes	BS degree
21. Sebastian	5	6	22	16	Scotland	Yes	Los Angeles	Yes	MA degree
22. Marianna	5	5	25	12	Northern Europe	Yes	Los Angeles	Yes	Some college
23. Joseph	3	2	20	17	Mexico	Yes	East Los Angeles	No, Yes	6th grade
24. Ann	4	1	21	17	Northern Europe	Yes	Southern California	Yes	MA degree in progress
25. Andrew	1	2	22	19	Britain	Yes	East Bay (Northern California)	No, Yes	PhD degree in progress
26. Mary	3	1	20	17	Africa-America	Yes	Southern California	Yes	High school
27. Leo	5	6	22	17	Mexico	Yes	Southern California	No	5th grade
28. Jacob	4	6	21	19	African American	Yes	Los Angeles	Yes	College
29. Susannah	4	2	22	15	Europe	Yes	Southern California	Yes	High school
30. Wheeler	4	7	22	17	France-Britain	No	Europe, Northern California	No	Some college

NOTE: Sexual orientation is explained on p. 174

Table A2 Comparison of Participants' Ethnic Groups With Class and Campus, 1992 (in Percentages)

Race	Participants	Respondents	Campus[c]
African-American	13.3	12.7	10.0
Asian	20.0	24.0[a]	30.0
Caucasian	43.3	37.9	33.0
Latino	23.3	12.7	15.0
Native American	0.0	5.0[b]	2.0

a. Includes one Persian Jew.
b. Includes three Native American/African Americans and one Native American-European American.
c. Berkeley Campus statistics for Fall 1992: Office of Institutional Research, Office of Student Research, June 1993.

Table A3 Age Distribution of Interview Participants

Age	18	19	20	21	22
Number	2	5	6	7	9
Percentage	6	16.67	20	23.33	30

greater interest in health and sexuality, indicated by taking the classes from which they were recruited, or the impact of course content might have had some impact on their experience, making them less likely to experience sexual health problems.

The measure of sexual orientation was based on a modified Kinsey scale presented in the vernacular, with a range from 1 (*exclusively heterosexual*) to 7 (*exclusively homosexual*):

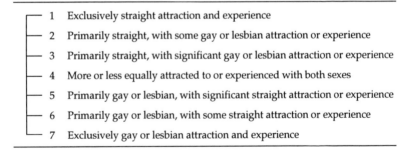

1	Exclusively straight attraction and experience
2	Primarily straight, with some gay or lesbian attraction or experience
3	Primarily straight, with significant gay or lesbian attraction or experience
4	More or less equally attracted to or experienced with both sexes
5	Primarily gay or lesbian, with significant straight attraction or experience
6	Primarily gay or lesbian, with some straight attraction or experience
7	Exclusively gay or lesbian attraction and experience

The Kinsey scale was used in this case because it is the most commonly understood and the fastest to complete, but it should be noted that two other scales exist that may better reflect the multidimensionality of sexuality, the Klein Grid and the Storms Scale (Udis-Kessler, 1992). The Klein Grid uses the Kinsey continuum to measure attraction, behavior, fantasies, emotional and social preference, self-identification, and lifestyle over the past, present, and intention for the future. The Storms scale approaches sexual orientation in much the same way that the BSRI measures gender role. On the Storms scale, one can be classified as heterosexual, homosexual, bisexual, or asexual.

The average sexual orientation rating for health education class survey respondents was 1.31 and was 1.72 for the 19 interview participants from that class (i.e., largely heterosexual). Because I was interested in comparing sexual negotiation across sexual orientation and the first recruitment turned up largely heterosexual students, I oversampled by recruiting additional participants from the sociology of sexuality class; the 11 interviewed from this class averaged 4.18. The average sexual orientation rating for the combined sample was then 2.36. Figure A1 compares sexual orientation, number of partners, and drinking behavior of the interview participants with the combined classes' responses on the RAQ, suggesting that interview participants were somewhat more sexually experienced than their peers. Although they claim to be a fairly abstinent lot, a good deal of unprotected sex occurs when the latter individuals are "drunk" or "drunk and horny." Sometimes, they are simply "stupid," overtaken by "hormones" or "in a hurry."

Not only do they overestimate their frequency of practicing safer sex (e.g. reporting having safer sex "always," but also reporting an STD or unplanned pregnancy), respondents don't share an understanding that safer sex refers to protection against STDs or HIV. Most identify it with condom use but with condom use for either STD prevention or pregnancy prevention. On the RAQ, I asked, "What exactly does safer sex entail for you? i.e., how does it alter your relationship; how do you make a specific behavior safer, or what behaviors do you avoid specifically because they are not safe?" Most responses were organized around using condoms and knowing one's partner. A minority wrote of getting tested for STDs, avoiding oral or anal sex, and of communicating with one's partner. A couple of people noted that condom use promoted communication for them and made sex more responsible. Several respondents mentioned using withdrawal as a safer sex method for both oral and genital intercourse. Knowing one's partner meant being in a "long-term relationship," presumably monogamous.

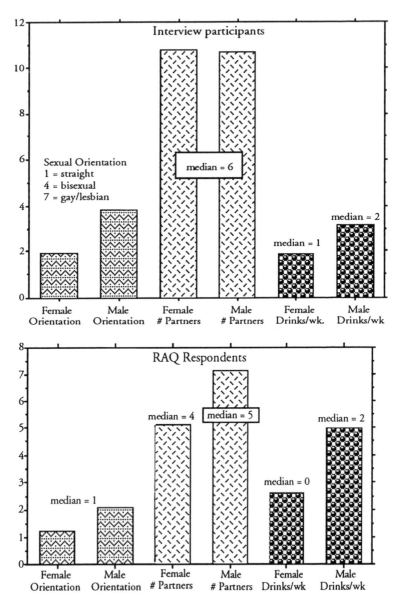

Figure A1. Sexual Orientation, Number of Lifetime Sexual Partners, and Average Number of Drinks per Week of Interview Participants (*n* = 30) and RAQ Respondents (*n* = 129)

Two most thoughtful responses came from virgins. One woman noted, "Safer sex not only means taking the precautions to prevent pregnancy, transfer of STDs and AIDS, but also making sure that sex is what both partners feel comfortable doing and talking about it." In response to the final question on the RAQ, "Is there anything else you would like me to know?" a man added, "We should be educated more about sex and relationships so that these experiences are more comfortable and pleasing." The most poignant quote on the RAQ came in response to this last item, from a gay man,

> It is important to realize that safer sex is not the same as safe sex: Although I was always militant in observing "safe sex" practices, I became infected with HIV—there are no guarantees. I feel confused and somewhat betrayed because despite taking precautions to avoid contact with body fluids every time, and having no knowledge of any "accidents" where something went wrong, it still happened. Looking back, I have a hard time figuring out how it happened. I just found out recently, so I'm still in a state of shock.

Responses such as this last emphasize the urgency of the need to find out exactly what people do, for as Bolton (1992) pointed out, there is much more to sexual activity than "sucking and fucking," knowledge of which may have helped this young man. Qualitative interviewing was an effective way to elicit sensitive information, one of the first in which interactionist theory has been used to guide the study of sexual interaction. One potential obstacle encountered in the application of interactionism to research on sexuality might be the possible effects of recall and the impossibility of direct observation. In this case, I was particularly experienced and comfortable discussing sexual topics; another researcher might not have the same combination of skill and luck. If interactionist understanding includes the construction of meaning about sexual negotiation, that meaning can well be created jointly in an interview situation. What might be learned through interpretive interactionism that would be less accessible by other methods? If we view sexual negotiation as a type of communication replete with symbols that can be interpreted, interactionism offers a viable method for understanding the dialectic of sexual relationships.

Note

1. Because initially I wasn't sure if the work would be externally funded, I wasn't sure what the amount would be. I believe strongly in paying research participants for their time, but if I'd been paying them out of my own pocket, it would have been less.

References

Abbey, A. (1982). Sex differences in attributions for friendly behavior: Do males misperceive females' friendliness? *Journal of Personality & Social Psychology, 42*(5), 830-838.

Abbey, A. (1991). Acquaintance rape and alcohol consumption on college campuses: How are they linked? *Journal of American College Health, 39*(4), 165-169.

Abramson, P. R. (1990). Sexual science: Emerging discipline or oxymoron? *The Journal of Sex Research, 27*(2), 147-165.

Abramson, P. R., & Herdt, G. (1990). The assessment of sexual practices relevant to the transmission of AIDS: A global perspective. *Journal of Sex Research, 27*(2), 215-232.

Ashcroft, D. M., Schlueter, D., & Thorton, G. (1991). *Safe-sex practices of rural area college students over a 12-year period.* Paper presented at the 99th Annual Convention of the American Psychological Association, San Francisco.

Baldwin, J. D., Whiteley, S., & Baldwin, J. I. (1992). The effect of ethnic group on sexual activities related to contraception and STDs. *Journal of Sex Research, 29*(2), 189-205.

Bachman, R. (1994). *Violence against women: A national crime victimization survey report.* Washington, DC: U.S. Department of Justice, Office of Justice Programs, Bureau of Justice Statistics.

Barkan, S., Deamant, C., Young, M., Stonis, L. F., Lucey, M., Wilson, T., Kilpatrick, S., Denenberg, R., & Melnick, S. (1996). *Sexual identity and behavior among women with female sexual partners: The Women's Interagency HIV Study (WIHS).* Eleventh International Conference on AIDS, Vancouver, BC, Canada.

Becker, H. S. (1961). *Boys in white: Student culture in medical school.* Chicago: University of Chicago Press.

Bell, S. T., Kuriloff, P. J., & Lottes, I. (1994). Understanding attributions of blame in stranger rape and date rape situations: An examination of gender, race, identification, and students' social perceptions of rape victims. *Journal of Applied Social Psychology, 24*(19), 1719-1734.

Bem, S. L. (1977). On the utility of alternative procedures for assessing psychological androgyny. *Journal of Consulting & Clinical Psychology, 45*(2), 196-205.

Bem, S. L. (1981). *Bem Sex-Role Inventory Professional Manual.* Palo Alto, California: Consulting Psychologists Press.

Bienenstock, A., & Epstein, N. (1979). Current adaptive challenges facing young females. In M. Sugar (Ed.), *Female adolescent development* (pp. 83-92). New York: Brunner/Mazel.

Blumer, H. (1969). *Symbolic interactionism: Perspective and method.* Englewood Cliffs, NJ: Prentice-Hall.

Bolton, R. (1992). Mapping terra incognita: Sex research for AIDS prevention: An urgent agenda for the 1990s. In G. Herdt & S. Lindenbaum (Eds.), *The time of AIDS: Social analysis, theory, and method* (pp. 124-158). Newbury Park, CA: Sage.

Canterbury, R. J., Grossman, S. J., & Lloyd, E. (1993). Drinking behavior and lifetime incidents of date rape among high school graduates upon entering college. *College Student Journal, 27*(1), 75-84.

Caplan, P. (Ed.). (1987). *The cultural construction of sexuality.* London: Tavistock.

Carrier, J. M. (1985). Mexican male bisexuality. *Journal of Homosexuality, 11*(1-2), 75-85.

Carroll, J. L., Volk, K. D., & Hyde, J. S. (1985). Differences between males and females in motives for engaging in sexual intercourse. *Archives of Sexual Behavior, 4*(2), 131-139.

CDC. (1993). *Preventing the sexual transmission of HIV and other STDs among a generation of young people 25 years of age and under: A Prevention Marketing Program.* Atlanta, GA: Centers for Disease Control.

Cobliner, W. G. (1988). The exclusion of intimacy in the sexuality of the contemporary college-age population. *Adolescence, 23*(89), 99-113.

Copenhaver, S., & Grauerholz, E. (1991). Sexual victimization among sorority women: Exploring the link between sexual violence and institutional practices. *Sex Roles, 24*(1/2), 31-41.

Deegan, M. J., & Hill, M. R. (Eds.). (1987). *Women and symbolic interaction.* Boston: Allen & Unwin.

Denzin, N. (1971, December). The logic of naturalistic inquiry. *Social Forces, 50,* 166-182.

Denzin, N. K. (1978). *The research act: A theoretical introduction to sociological methods* (2nd ed.). New York: McGraw-Hill.

Denzin, N. K. (1989). *Interpretive interactionism.* Newbury Park, CA: Sage.

Denzin, N. K. (1992). *Symbolic interactionism and cultural studies: The politics of interpretation.* Cambridge, MA: Blackwell.

Denzin, N. K., & Lincoln, Y. S. (Eds.). (1994). *Handbook of qualitative research* (1st ed.). Thousand Oaks, CA: Sage.

Division of STD Prevention. (1995). *Sexually transmitted disease surveillance, 1994.* Washington, DC: U.S. Department of Health and Human Services, Public Health Service.

Dunne, M. P., Donald, M., Lucke, J., Nilsson, R., Ballard, R., & Raphael, B. (1994). Age-related increase in sexual behaviors and decrease in regular condom use among adolescents in Australia. *International Journal of STD & AIDS, 5,* 41-47.

Earle, J. R., & Perricone, P. J. (1986). Premarital sexuality: A ten-year study of attitudes and behavior on a small university campus. *The Journal of Sex Research, 22*(3), 304-310

Ehrhardt, A. A. (1996). Editorial: Our view of adolescent sexuality—A focus on risk behavior without the development context. *American Journal of Public Health, 86*(11), 1523-1525.

Fine, M. (1988). Sexuality, schooling, and adolescent females: The missing discourse of desire. *Harvard Educational Review, 58*(1), 29-53.

Fine, M. (1994). Dis-stance and other stances: Negotiations of power inside feminist research. In A. Gitlin (Ed.). *Power and method: Political activism and educational research* (pp. 13-35). New York: Routledge.

Foley, L. A., Evancic, C., Karnik, K., King, J., & Parks, A. (1995). Date rape: Effects of race of assailant and victim and gender of subjects on perceptions. *Journal of Black Psychology, 21*(1), 6-18.

Foucault, M. (1980). *The history of sexuality.* New York: Random House.

Foucault, M. (1984). *Histoire de la Sexualité 3: Le Souci de Soi.* Paris: Gallimard.

Frankenberg, R. (1992). The other who is also the same: The relevance of epidemics in space and time for prevention of HIV infection. *International Journal of Health Services, 22*(1), 73-78.

Frankenberg, R. J. (1994). The impact of HIV/AIDS on concepts relating to risk and culture within British community epidemiology: Candidates or targets for prevention? *Social Science and Medicine, 38*(10), 1325-1335.

Gagnon, J. H. (1977). *Human sexualities.* Glenview, IL: Scott, Foresman.

Gagnon, J. H. (1992). Epidemics and researchers: AIDS and the practice of social studies. In G. Herdt & S. Lindenbaum (Eds.), *The time of AIDS: Social analysis, theory, and method* (pp. 27-40). Newbury Park, CA: Sage.

Gagnon, J. H., & Simon, W. (1973). *Sexual conduct: The social sources of human sexuality.* Chicago: Aldine.

Gaies, L. A., Sacco, W. P., & Becker, J. A. (1991). *Cognitions related to high risk sexual behavior.* Paper presented at the 99th Annual Convention of the American Psychological Association, San Francisco.

Gilbert, N., Muehlenhard, C. L., Highby, B. J., Phelps, J. L. (1997). Rape: Are rape statistics exaggerated? In M. R. Walsh (Ed.), *Men, women, and gender: Ongoing debates* (pp. 233-246). New Haven, CT: Yale University Press.

Gilligan, C. (1982). *In a different voice.* Cambridge, MA: Harvard University Press.

Glaser, B. G., & Strauss, A. L. (1971). *Status passage.* Chicago: Aldine, Atherton.

Goffman, E. (1961). *Asylums: Essays on the social situation of mental patients and other inmates.* Garden City, NY: Anchor.

Gold, J., Li, Y., & Kaldor, J. M. (1994, December 19). Premature mortality in Australia 1983-1992, the first decade of the AIDS epidemic. *Medical Journal of Australia, 161*, 656-656.

Gold, R. S., & Skinner, M. J. (1992). Situational factors and thought processes associated with unprotected intercourse in young gay men. *AIDS, 6*(9), 1021-1030.

Gordon, T. E. (1996). The need for adolescent health education and training among health professionals [Letter]. *American Journal of Public Health, 86*(6), 889.

Grimley, D., Prochaska, J. O., Velicer, W. F., Blais, L. M., & DiClemente, C. C. (1994). The transtheoretical model of change. In T. M. Brinthaupt & R. P. Lipka (Eds.), *Changing the self: Philosophies, techniques, and experiences* (pp. 201-207). Albany, NY: State University of New York Press.

Grimley, D. M., Riley, G. E., Bellis, J. M., & Prochaska, J. O. (1993). Assessing the stages of change and decision-making for contraceptive use for the prevention of pregnancy, sexually transmitted diseases, and Acquired Immunodeficiency Syndrome. *Health Education Quarterly, 20*(4), 455-470.

Hein, K. (1988). *AIDS in adolescence: A rationale for concern* (Working paper). New York: Carnegie Council on Adolescent Development.

Herdt, G., & Boxer, A. M. (1991). Ethnographic issues in the study of AIDS. *Journal of Sex Research, 28*(2), 171-187.

Herdt, G., & Lindenbaum, S. (Eds.). (1992). *The time of AIDS: Social analysis, theory and method.* Newbury Park, CA: Sage.

Hesse-Biber, S., Dupuis, P., & Kinder, T. S. (1991). HyperRESEARCH™: A computer program for the analysis of qualitative data with an emphasis on hypothesis testing and multimedia analysis. *Qualitative Sociology, 14*(4), 289-306.

Holcomb, D. R., Sarvela, P. D., Sondag, A. K., & Holcomb, L. H. (1993). An evaluation of a mixed-gender date rape prevention workshop. *Journal of American College Health, 41*(4), 159-164.

Holland, J., Ramazanoglu, C., & Scott, S. (1990). AIDS: From panic stations to power relations—Sociological perspectives and problems. *Sociology, 25*(3), 499-518.

Holland, J., Ramazanoglu, C., Scott, S., Sharpe, S., & Thomson, R. (1990). *"Don't die of ignorance—I nearly died of embarrassment": Condoms in context.* London: Tufnell.

Holland, J., Ramazanoglu, C., Scott, S., Sharpe, S., & Thomson, R. (1991). Between embarrassment and trust: Young women and the diversity of condom use. In P. Aggleton, G. Hart, & P. Davies (Eds.), *AIDS: Responses, interventions and care* (pp. 127-148). London: Falmer.

Holland, J., Ramazanoglu, C., Sharpe, S., & Thomson, R. (1991, March). *Pressured pleasure: Young women and the negotiation of sexual boundaries.* Paper presented at the British Sociological Association Annual Conference, Manchester, UK.

Holland, J., Ramazanoglu, C., Sharpe, S., & Thomson, R. (1994). Achieving masculine sexuality: Young men's strategies for managing vulnerability. In L. Doyal, J. Naidoo, & T. Wilton (Eds.), *AIDS: Setting a feminist agenda* (pp. 122-148). London: Taylor & Francis.

Huang, K., & Uba, L. (1992). Premarital sexual behavior among Chinese college students in the United States. *Archives of Sexual Behavior, 21*(3), 227-240.

Jackson, T. L. (1991). A university athletic department's rape and assault experiences. *Journal of College Student Development, 32*(1), 77-78.

James, N. J., Bignell, C. J., & Gillies, P. A. (1991). The reliability of self-reported sexual behavior. *AIDS, 5,* 333-336.

Keller, J. F., Elliot, S. S., & Gunberg, E. (1982). Premarital sexual intercourse among single college students: A discriminant analysis. *Sex Roles, 8*(1), 21-32.

Kemp, G., Jones, M., Kellogg, T., Martinez, T., Lakhana, P., & Storey, S. (1993). *HIV seroprevalance and risk behaviors among lesbians and bisexual women: The 1993 San Francisco/Berkeley Women's Study.* San Francisco: San Francisco Department of Public Health, Surveillance Branch, AIDS Office.

Kippax, S., Crawford, J., & Waldby, C. (1994). Heterosexuality, masculinity and HIV. *AIDS, 8*(Suppl. 1), S315-S323.

Kippax, S., Crawford, J., Waldby, C., & Benton, P. (1990). Women negotiating heterosex: Implications for AIDS prevention. *Women's Studies International Forum, 13*(6), 533-542.

Kitzinger, C. (1987). *The social construction of lesbianism.* London: Sage.

Koralewski, M. A., & Conger, J. C. (1992). The assessment of social skills among sexually coercive college males. *Journal of Sex Research, 29*(2), 169-188.

Koss, M. P. (1992). Defending date rape. *Journal of Interpersonal Violence, 7*(1), 122-126.

Lear, D. (1990). AIDS in the African press. *International Quarterly of Community Health Education, 10*(3), 253-264.

Lear, D. (1994). *Sexual communication in the age of AIDS* (Doctoral dissertation, University of California, Berkeley, University Microfilms No. 9528699).

Leigh, B. C. (1989). Reasons for having and avoiding sex: Gender, sexual orientation, and relationship to sexual behavior. *Journal of Sex Research, 26*(2), 199-209.

Lenihan, G. O., Rawlins, M. E., Eberly, C. G., & Buckley, B. (1992). Gender differences in rape supportive attitudes before and after a date rape education intervention. *Journal of College Student Development, 33*(4), 331-338.

Lever, J., Kanouse, D. E., Rogers, W. H., & Hertz, R. (1992). Behavior patterns and sexual identity of bisexual males. *Journal of Sex Research, 29*(2), 141-167.

Levine, M. P. (1992). The implications of constructionist theory for social research on the AIDS epidemic among gay men. In G. Herdt & S. Lindenbaum (Eds.), *The time of AIDS: Social analysis, theory, and method* (pp. 185-198). Newbury Park, CA: Sage.

Leviton, L. C. (1989). Theoretical foundations of AIDS prevention programs. In R. O. Valdiserri (Ed.), *Preventing AIDS: The design of effective programs* (pp. 42-90). New Brunswick, NJ: Rutgers University.

Lowy, E., & Ross, M. W. (1994). "It'll never happen to me": Gay men's beliefs, perceptions and folk constructions of sexual risk. *AIDS Education and Prevention, 6*(6), 467-482.

Lucke, J. (1994). *A study of the influence of contraceptive use on the sexual risk practices of young women: Implications for practice.* Brisbane, QLD, Austalia: National Centre for HIV Social Research, University of Queensland.

Lucke, J., Dunne, M., Donald, M., & Raphael, B. (1993). Knowledge of STDs and perceived risk of infection: A study of Australian youth. *Venereology, 6*(3), 57-63.

Maticka-Tyndale, E. (1991a). Modification of sexual activities in the era of AIDS: A trend analysis of adolescent sexual activities. *Youth & Society, 23*(1), 31-49.

Maticka-Tyndale, E. (1991b). Sexual scripts and AIDS prevention: Variations in adherence to safer-sex guidelines by heterosexual adolescents. *Journal of Sex Research, 28*(1), 45-66.

McCall, M. M., & Wittner, J. (1990). The good news about life history. In H. S. Becker & M. M. McCall (Eds.), *Symbolic interaction and cultural studies.* Chicago: University of Chicago Press.

Mead, G. H. (1934). *Mind, self and society.* Chicago: University of Chicago Press.

Mead, G. H. (1982). *The individual and the social self.* Chicago: University of Chicago Press.

Middleton, W., Harris, P., & Hollely, C. (1994). Condom use by heterosexual students: Justifications for unprotected intercourse. *Health Education Journal, 53,* 147-154.

Midwinter, D. Y. (1992). Rule prescriptions for initial male-female interaction. *Sex Roles, 26*(5/6), 161-173.

Mills, C. S., & Granoff, B. J. (1992). Date and acquaintance rape among a sample of college students. *Social Work, 37*(6), 504-509.

Moore, S., & Rosenthal, D. (1993). *Sexuality in adolescence.* London: Routledge.

Moore, S. M., & Rosenthal, D. A. (1991). Condoms and coitus: Adolescents' attitudes to AIDS and safe sex behavior. *Journal of Adolescence, 14,* 211-227.

Morton, M., Nelson, L., Walsh, C., Zimmerman, S., & Coe, R. M. (1996). Evaluation of a HIV/AIDS education program for adolescents. *Journal of Community Health, 21*(1), 23-35.

Muehlenhard, C. L. (1988). Misinterpreted dating behaviors and the risk of date rape. *Social and Clinical Psychology, 6*(1), 20-37.

Muehlenhard, C. L., & Falcon, P. L. (1990). Men's heterosocial skill and attitudes toward women as predictors of verbal sexual coercion and forceful rape. *Sex Roles, 23*(5/6), 241-259.

Muehlenhard, C. L., & McCoy, M. L. (1991). Double standard/double bind: The sexual double standard and women's communication about sex. *Psychology of Women Quarterly, 15,* 447-461.

Oakley, A. (1981). Interviewing women: A contradiction in terms. In H. Roberts (Ed.), *Doing feminist research* (pp. 30-61). London: Routledge & Kegan Paul.

Office of National AIDS Policy. (1996). *Youth & HIV/AIDS: An American agenda.* Washington, DC: National AIDS Fund.

Ogletree, R. J. (1993). Sexual coercion experience and help-seeking behavior of college women. *Journal of American College Health, 41*(4), 149-153.

Padilla, E. R., & O'Grady, K. E. (1987). Sexuality among Mexican Americans: A case of sexual stereotyping. *Journal of Personality and Social Psychology, 52*(1), 5-10.

Paglia, C. (1990, December 14). Madonna—Finally, a real feminist. *New York Times,* pp. A21, A39.

Paglia, C. (1993, January-February). It's a jungle out there, so get used to it! *Utne Reader, 55,* 61-65.

Parker, R. G. (1992). Sexual diversity, cultural analysis, and AIDS education in Brazil. In G. Herdt & S. Lindenbaum (Eds.), *The time of AIDS: Social analysis, theory, and method* (pp. 225-242). Newbury Park, CA: Sage.

Parker, R. G., & Carballo, M. (1990). Qualitative research on homosexual and bisexual behavior relevant to HIV/AIDS. *Journal of Sex Research, 27*(4), 497-525.

Parker, R. G., & Gagnon, J. H. (Eds.). (1995). *Conceiving sexuality: Approaches to sex research in a postmodern world.* New York: Routledge.

Parker, R. G., Herdt, G., & Carballo, M. (1991). Sexual culture, HIV transmission and AIDS research. *Journal of Sex Research, 28*(1), 77-98.

Paul, E. L., & White, K. M. (1990). The development of intimate relationships in late adolescence. *Adolescence, 25*(98), 375-399.

Pennbridge, J. N., Freese, T. E., & MacKenzie, R. G. (1992). High-risk behaviors among male street youth in Hollywood, California. *AIDS Education & Prevention*(Suppl.), 24-33.

Plummer, K. (1975). *Sexual stigma.* London: Routledge.

Plummer, K. (Ed.). (1995). *Telling sexual stories: Power, change and social worlds.* London: Routledge.

Porter, J. F., Critelli, J. W., & Tang, C. S. (1992). Sexual and aggressive motives in sexually aggressive college males. *Archives of Sexual Behavior, 21*(5), 457-468.

Romer, D., Black, M., Ricardo, I., Feigelman, S., Kaljee, L., Galbraith, J., Nesbit, R., Hornik, R. C., & Stanton, B. (1994). Social influences on the sexual behavior of youth at risk for HIV exposure. *American Journal of Public Health, 84*(6), 977-984.

Roscoe, B., & Kruger, T. L. (1990). AIDS: Late adolescents' knowledge and its influence on sexual behavior. *Adolescence, 25*(97), 39-48.

Roscoe, B., & Peterson, K. L. (1984). Older adolescents: A self-report of engagement in developmental tasks. *Adolescence, 19*(74), 391-396.

Rosenstock, I. M. (1974). The Health Belief Model and preventive health behavior. *Health Education Monographs, 2*(4), 354-386.

Rotheram-Borus, M. J., Meyer-Bahlbur, H. F., Rosario, M., & Koopman, C. (1992). Lifetime sexual behaviors among predominantly minority male runaways and gay/bisexual adolescents in New York City. *AIDS Education & Prevention*(Suppl.), 34-42.

Rowe, P. M. (1996). Case for behavioral studies for AIDS prevention. *Lancet, 347*(9002), 750.

Sabogal, F., Sandlin, G., Reyes, R., Aguirre, V., Bregman, G., & Kemp, G. (1991). *San Francisco Latino gay/bisexual males' HIV knowledge, attitudes, and behaviors.* Paper presented at the 99th Annual Convention of the American Psychological Association, San Francisco.

Sanday, P. R. (1990). *Fraternity gang rape: Sex, brotherhood, and privilege on campus.* New York: New York University Press.

Sawyer, R. G., Desmond, S. M., & Lucke, G. M. (1993). Sexual communication and the college student: Implications for date rape. *Health Values: The Journal of Health Behavior, Education, and Promotion, 17*(4), 11-20.

Schuster, M. A., Bell, R. M., & Kanouse, D. E. (1996). The sexual practices of adolescent virgins: Genital sexual activities of high school students who have never had vaginal intercourse. *American Journal of Public Health, 86*(11), 1570-1576.

Schwant, T. A. (1994). Constructivist, interpretivist approaches to human inquiry. In N. K. Denzin & Y. S. Lincoln (Eds.), *Handbook of qualitative research* (pp. 118-137). Thousand Oaks, CA: Sage.

Schwartz, H., & Jacobs, J. (1979). *Qualitative sociology.* New York: Free Press.

Scott, A., & Griffin, H. (1989). *Concept testing the Dundee "Condoms in AIDS prevention" initiative.* Glasgow, UK: Tayside Health Board, Advertising Research Unit, University of Strathclyde.

Sheldon-Keller, A., Lloyd-McGarvey, E., West, M., & Canterbury, R. J. (1994). Attachment and assessment of blame in date rape scenarios. *Social Behavior & Personality, 22*(4), 313-318.

Shotland, R. L., & Hunter, B. A. (1995). Women's "token resistant" and compliant sexual behaviors are related to uncertain sexual intentions and rape. *Personality & Social Psychology Bulletin, 21*(3), 226-236.

Skidmore, W. (1979). *Theoretical thinking in sociology.* Cambridge, UK: Cambridge University Press.

Spigner, C. (1989-1990). Sociology of AIDS within Black communities: Theoretical considerations. *International Quarterly of Community Health Education, 10*(4), 285-296.

Taylor, C. L., & Lourea, D. (1992). HIV prevention: A dramaturgical analysis and practical guide to creating safer sex interventions [Special issue: Rethinking AIDS prevention: Cultural approaches]. *Medical Anthropology, 14*(2-4), 243-284.

Trocki, K. F. (1992). Patterns of sexuality and risky sexuality in the general population of a California county. *Journal of Sex Research, 29*(1), 85-94.

Udis-Kessler, A. (1992). Appendix: Notes on the Kinsey scale and other measures of sexuality. In E. R. Weise (Ed.), *Closer to home: Bisexuality and feminism* (pp. 311-318). Seattle: Seal.

Ulin, P. R. (1992). African women and AIDS: Negotiating behavioral change. *Social Science and Medicine, 34*(1), 63-73.

Vance, C. S. (Ed.). (1984). *Pleasure and danger: Exploring female sexuality.* Boston: Routledge & Kegan Paul.

Vance, C. S. (1991). Anthropology rediscovers sexuality: A theoretical comment. *Social Science and Medicine, 33*(8), 875-884.

Vidich, A. J., & Lyman, S. M. (1994). Qualitative methods: Their history in sociology and anthropology. In N. K. Denzin & Y. S. Lincoln (Eds.), *Handbook of qualitative research* (pp. 23-59). Thousand Oaks, CA: Sage.

Weeks, J. (1985). *Sexuality and its discontents.* London: Routledge & Kegan Paul.

White, S. D., & DeBlassie, R. R. (1992). Adolescent sexual behavior. *Adolescence, 27*(105), 183-191.

Wight, D. (1992). Impediments to safer heterosexual sex: A review of research with young people. *AIDS Care, 4*(1), 11-21.

Wyatt, G. E. (1989). Reexamining factors predicting Afro-American and White American women's age at first coitus. *Archives of Sexual Behavior, 18*(4), 271-298.

Wyatt, G. E., & Lyons-Rowe, S. (1990). African American women's sexual satisfaction as a dimension of their sex roles. *Sex Roles, 22*(7/8), 509-524.

Yankelovich, D. (1974). *The new morality profile of American youth in the seventies.* New York: McGraw-Hill.

Name Index

Subject Index

About the Author

Dana Lear teaches Community Health at the University of Sydney, Australia. She completed her DrPH in the department of community health education at the University of California, Berkeley in 1994. She is currently researching the social construction of sexuality among young men in Brisbane and Sydney. Dr. Lear has also published on HIV in Africa and women's mental health issues. She has worked in community health in Canada, Jamaica, the U.S., West Africa and Australia. Her own experiences negotiating relationships in the '90s led her to wonder how people who have grown up in an era of feminism and AIDS awareness resolve these issues.